# APPLIED SOCIOLOGY FOR NURSING
## and Allied Health Sciences

# APPLIED SOCIOLOGY FOR NURSING
## and Allied Health Sciences

**Second Edition**

**Tara Madhusudan**
MA (Sociology) Diploma in Higher Education (Mumbai University)
*Formerly*
Lecturer in Sociology
RV College of Nursing and
RV College of Physiotherapy
Bengaluru, Karnataka, India

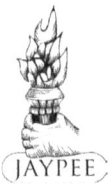

**JAYPEE BROTHERS MEDICAL PUBLISHERS**
*The Health Sciences Publisher*
New Delhi | London

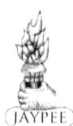 **Jaypee Brothers Medical Publishers (P) Ltd**

**Headquarters**
Jaypee Brothers Medical Publishers (P) Ltd
EMCA House, 23/23-B
Ansari Road, Daryaganj
New Delhi 110 002, India
Landline: +91-11-23272143
+91-11-23272703, +91-11-23282021
+91-11-23245672
Email: jaypee@jaypeebrothers.com

**Corporate Office**
Jaypee Brothers Medical Publishers (P) Ltd
4838/24, Ansari Road, Daryaganj
New Delhi 110 002, India
Phone: +91-11-43574357
Fax: +91-11-43574314
Email: jaypee@jaypeebrothers.com

**Overseas Office**
J.P. Medical Ltd
83 Victoria Street, London
SW1H 0HW (UK)
Phone: +44 20 3170 8910
Email: info@jpmedpub.com

**EU GPSR** Authorised Representative
Logos Europe, 9 rue Nicolas Poussin
17000, La Rochelle, France
Phone: +33 (0) 6 67 93 73 78
E-mail: Contact@logoseurope.eu

Website: www.jaypeebrothers.com
Website: www.jaypeedigital.com

© 2023, Jaypee Brothers Medical Publishers

The views and opinions expressed in this book are solely those of the original contributor(s)/author(s) and do not necessarily represent those of editor(s) and publisher of the book.

All rights reserved. No part of this publication may be reproduced, stored or transmitted in any form or by any means, electronic, mechanical, photocopying, recording or otherwise, without the prior permission in writing of the publishers.

All brand names and product names used in this book are trade names, service marks, trademarks or registered trademarks of their respective owners. The publisher is not associated with any product or vendor mentioned in this book.

Medical knowledge and practice change constantly. This book is designed to provide accurate, authoritative information about the subject matter in question. However, readers are advised to check the most current information available on procedures included and check information from the manufacturer of each product to be administered, to verify the recommended dose, formula, method and duration of administration, adverse effects and contraindications. It is the responsibility of the practitioner to take all appropriate safety precautions. Neither the publisher nor the author(s)/editor(s) assume any liability for any injury and/or damage to persons or property arising from or related to use of material in this book.

This book is sold on the understanding that the publisher is not engaged in providing professional medical services. If such advice or services are required, the services of a competent medical professional should be sought.

Every effort has been made where necessary to contact holders of copyright to obtain permission to reproduce copyright material. If any have been inadvertently overlooked, the publisher will be pleased to make the necessary arrangements at the first opportunity.

**Inquiries for bulk sales may be solicited at:** jaypee@jaypeebrothers.com

*Applied Sociology for Nursing and Allied Health Sciences*

First Edition: 2011
Second Edition: **2023**
ISBN: 978-93-5465-669-9

# APPLIED SOCIOLOGY FOR NURSING
## and Allied Health Sciences

**Second Edition**

**Tara Madhusudan**
MA (Sociology) Diploma in Higher Education (Mumbai University)
*Formerly*
Lecturer in Sociology
RV College of Nursing and
RV College of Physiotherapy
Bengaluru, Karnataka, India

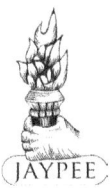

**JAYPEE BROTHERS MEDICAL PUBLISHERS**
*The Health Sciences Publisher*
New Delhi | London

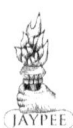 **Jaypee Brothers Medical Publishers (P) Ltd**

**Headquarters**
Jaypee Brothers Medical Publishers (P) Ltd
EMCA House, 23/23-B
Ansari Road, Daryaganj
New Delhi 110 002, India
Landline: +91-11-23272143
+91-11-23272703, +91-11-23282021
+91-11-23245672
Email: jaypee@jaypeebrothers.com

**Corporate Office**
Jaypee Brothers Medical Publishers (P) Ltd
4838/24, Ansari Road, Daryaganj
New Delhi 110 002, India
Phone: +91-11-43574357
Fax: +91-11-43574314
Email: jaypee@jaypeebrothers.com

**Overseas Office**
J.P. Medical Ltd
83 Victoria Street, London
SW1H 0HW (UK)
Phone: +44 20 3170 8910
Email: info@jpmedpub.com

**EU GPSR** Authorised Representative
Logos Europe, 9 rue Nicolas Poussin
17000, La Rochelle, France
Phone: +33 (0) 6 67 93 73 78
E-mail: Contact@logoseurope.eu

Website: www.jaypeebrothers.com
Website: www.jaypeedigital.com

© 2023, Jaypee Brothers Medical Publishers

The views and opinions expressed in this book are solely those of the original contributor(s)/author(s) and do not necessarily represent those of editor(s) and publisher of the book.

All rights reserved. No part of this publication may be reproduced, stored or transmitted in any form or by any means, electronic, mechanical, photocopying, recording or otherwise, without the prior permission in writing of the publishers.

All brand names and product names used in this book are trade names, service marks, trademarks or registered trademarks of their respective owners. The publisher is not associated with any product or vendor mentioned in this book.

Medical knowledge and practice change constantly. This book is designed to provide accurate, authoritative information about the subject matter in question. However, readers are advised to check the most current information available on procedures included and check information from the manufacturer of each product to be administered, to verify the recommended dose, formula, method and duration of administration, adverse effects and contraindications. It is the responsibility of the practitioner to take all appropriate safety precautions. Neither the publisher nor the author(s)/editor(s) assume any liability for any injury and/or damage to persons or property arising from or related to use of material in this book.

This book is sold on the understanding that the publisher is not engaged in providing professional medical services. If such advice or services are required, the services of a competent medical professional should be sought.

Every effort has been made where necessary to contact holders of copyright to obtain permission to reproduce copyright material. If any have been inadvertently overlooked, the publisher will be pleased to make the necessary arrangements at the first opportunity.

**Inquiries for bulk sales may be solicited at:** jaypee@jaypeebrothers.com

*Applied Sociology for Nursing and Allied Health Sciences*

First Edition: 2011

Second Edition: **2023**

ISBN: 978-93-5465-669-9

# Dedicated to

*My parents*
*Late Shri Dwaraknath Woody*
*and*
*Late Smt Meenakshi Woody*

# Preface to the Second Edition

Sociology is the science of society which has a very wide scope. It studies all aspects of man as a social being like his relationships, the groups he forms, his behaviors and cultures. Man needs to be treated not only as a biological being, but also as a social, psychological, cultural and rational being. The study of this subject gives the health care professionals a holistic understanding for treating the patients.

This book attempts to give a better understanding of man and society by dealing with the processes of socialization, social processes, social group like family and marriage, communities to which he belongs like rural, urban and regional, stratification processes, such as caste, class and race in the society, population, social problems existing in the society and social changes.

**Tara Madhusudan**

# Preface to the First Edition

Sociology is the science of society. It is the scientific study of human beings, their relationships, the groups they form and their behavior and culture. Man needs to be treated not only as a biological being but also as a social, cultural and rational being. Study of Sociology becomes necessary for the health care professionals as they have to deal with human beings. It will give them a holistic understanding of the patients for the treatment.

This book is written to serve as a textbook for the graduate courses of nursing and allied health sciences. The book covers the syllabi prescribed by the Nursing Council of India. I am enthused to bring out this book as I am presently teaching the subject for the above-mentioned courses.

**Tara Madhusudan**

# Acknowledgments

I wish to thank my son, Mr WM Shashank for assisting me in proofreading of the manuscript and valuable suggestions.

I thank M/s Jaypee Brothers Medical Publishers (P) Ltd, New Delhi, India and in particular their Bengaluru branch manager and his staff for the coordinating efforts in bringing out this publication.

# Contents

1. **An Introduction to Sociology** ................................................. 1
   Definition  3
   Nature of Sociology  4
   Scope of Sociology  6
   Sociology and other Social Sciences  7
   Methods of Social Investigations  12
   Importance of Sociology  15
   Social Factors in Health and Disease Situations  19

2. **Man and Society** ........................................................................ 24
   Definition  24
   Community and Association  27
   Process of Socialization  30
   Agencies of Socialization  34

3. **Culture** ........................................................................................ 39
   Definition  39
   Nature or Characteristics of Culture  40
   Evolution or Development of Culture  41
   Diversity and Uniformity of Culture  42
   Functions of Culture  44
   Cultural Factors in Health and Disease  45

4. **Social Processes** ....................................................................... 48
   Definition  49
   Forms of Social Processes  50
   Associative or Conjunctive Social Processes  50
   Types of Cooperation  51
   Role of Cooperation in Social Life or
   Importance of Cooperation  52
   Accommodation  52
   Forms or Methods of Accommodation  54
   Role of Accommodation  57
   Assimilation  57

Competition *61*
Nature and Characteristics of Competition *62*
Nature and Characteristics of Conflict *66*
Role of Conflict *68*

**5. Social Groups** .......................................................................... **73**
Meaning *74*
Characteristics of Social Groups *74*
Classification of Social Groups *76*
CH Cooley's Classification of Social Groups *78*
Ethnocentrism *83*

**6. Family and Marriage** ............................................................. **94**
Family *94*
Characteristics of the Family *95*
Functions of the Family *96*
Problems of the Modern Family *100*
Types or Forms of Family *101*
Indian Family—The Joint Family System *104*
Merits and Demerits of the Joint Family System *106*
Disintegration of the Joint Family System *108*
Family Welfare Services *113*
Marriage *114*
Forms of Marriage *114*
Marriage and Family Problems in India *116*
Influence of Family on the Individual's Health *118*

**7. Rural Community** ................................................................. **122**
The Rural or Village Community *122*
Characteristics of the Indian Village *124*
Change in Indian Rural Life *126*
Community Development Project and Planning *128*
Problems of Villages or Rural Community *129*

**8. Urban and Regional Community** ....................................... **132**
Urban—The Growth in the Cities *132*
Features of Urban Community *133*
City Community in India *135*
Urban-Rural Contrast *135*
Major Urban Problems *137*
The Regional Community *139*

## 9. Social Stratification ............................................................. 141
Class and Caste  *141*
The Indian Caste System  *142*
Origin of Caste System  *147*
Caste in India Today  *148*
Features of Caste System in India  *149*
Social Mobility  *152*

## 10. Social System ..................................................................... 154
Meaning  *154*
Principal Types of Social System  *156*
Role and Status  *158*

## 11. Race .................................................................................. 164
Definition  *164*
Determinants of Race  *165*
Races in India  *166*

## 12. Population ......................................................................... 168
Society and Population  *168*
Distribution of Population  *169*
Malthusian Theory of Population  *170*
Population Explosion in India  *170*
Evil Effects or Consequences of Over-Population  *171*

## 13. Social Control .................................................................... 174
Meaning  *174*
Definitions  *174*
Types of Social Control  *175*
Norms and Values  *177*
Folkways and Mores  *179*
The Social Role of Custom  *183*
Fashion  *186*
The Social Role of Fashion in the Modern Society  *188*

## 14. Social Problems ................................................................. 190
Social Disorganization  *190*
Social Problems  *193*
Major Social Problems  *194*
Unemployment  *196*
Beggary  *197*
Illiteracy  *199*

Contents

Housing  *200*
Food Supplies  *201*
Prostitution  *203*
Rights of Women and Children  *204*
Vulnerable Groups  *205*
Handicapped  *206*
Minority and Other Marginalized Groups  *207*
Delinquency and Crime  *208*
Child Labor-Child Abuse  *210*
Child Abuse  *211*
Alcoholism  *213*
Substance Abuse or Drug Abuse  *214*
Social Welfare Programs in India  *217*

15. **Social Change** ............................................................................. **223**
Definition  *223*
Nature of Social Change  *224*
Factors Influencing Social Change  *225*
Theories of Social Change  *228*
Role of Nurse as Agents of Social Change  *230*

16. **Social Security and Social Work** ......................................... **232**
Social Security  *232*
Social Security Legislations in India  *233*
Social work  *233*

*Bibliography* ................................................................................................ *235*
*Index* ............................................................................................................. *237*

# INC Syllabus

## APPLIED SOCIOLOGY

**PLACEMENT:** I SEMESTER

**THEORY:** 3 Credits (60 hours)

**DESCRIPTION:** This course is designed to enable the students to develop understanding about basic concepts of sociology and its application in personal and community life, health, illness and nursing.

**COMPETENCIES:** On completion of the course, the students will be able to:
- Identify the scope and significance of sociology in nursing.
- Apply the knowledge of social structure and different culture in a society in identifying social needs of sick clients.
- Identify the impact of culture on health and illness.
- Develop understanding about types of family, marriage and its legislation.
- Identify different types of caste, class, social change and its influence on health and health practices.
- Develop understanding about social organization and disorganization and social problems in India.
- Integrate the knowledge of clinical sociology and its uses in crisis intervention.

# INC Syllabus

## COURSE OUTLINE
### T – Theory

| Unit | Time (Hrs) | Learning Outcomes | Content | Teaching/Learning Activities | Assessment Methods |
|---|---|---|---|---|---|
| I. | 1 (T) | Describe the scope and significance of sociology in nursing | **Introduction**<br>• Definition, nature and scope of sociology<br>• Significance of sociology in nursing | • Lecture<br>• Discussion | • Essay<br>• Short answer |
| II. | 15 (T) | Describe the individualization, Groups, processes of socialization, social change and its importance | **Social structure**<br>• Basic concept of society, community, association and institution<br>• Individual and society<br>• Personal disorganization<br>• Social group—meaning, characteristics, and classification<br>• Social processes—definition and forms, cooperation, competition, conflict, accommodation, assimilation, isolation<br>• Socialization—characteristics, process, agencies of socialization<br>• Social change—nature, process and role of nurse | • Lecture cum Discussion | • Essay<br>• Short answer<br>• Objective type |

*Contd...*

*Contd...*

| Unit | Time (Hrs) | Learning Outcomes | Content | Teaching/ Learning Activities | Assessment Methods |
|---|---|---|---|---|---|
| | | | • Structure and characteristics of urban, rural and tribal community<br>• Major health problems in urban, rural and tribal communities<br>• Importance of social structure in nursing profession | | |
| III | 8 (T) | Describe culture and its impact on health and disease | **Culture**<br>• Nature, characteristic and evolution of culture<br>• Diversity and uniformity of culture<br>• Difference between culture and civilization<br>• Culture and socialization<br>• Transcultural society<br>• Culture, modernization and its impact on health and disease | • Lecture<br>• Panel discussion | • Essay<br>• Short answer |
| IV | 8 (T) | Explain family, marriage and legislation related to marriage | **Family and Marriage**<br>• Family—characteristics, basic need, types and functions of family<br>• Marriage—forms of marriage, social custom relating to marriage and importance of marriage<br>• Legislation on Indian marriage and family.<br>• Influence of marriage and family on health and health practices | • Lecture | • Essay<br>• Short answer<br>• Case study report |

*Contd...*

Contd...

| Unit | Time (Hrs) | Learning Outcomes | Content | Teaching/ Learning Activities | Assessment Methods |
|---|---|---|---|---|---|
| V | 8 (T) | Explain different types of caste and classes in society and its influence on health | **Social stratification**<br>- Introduction—Characteristics and forms of stratification<br>- Function of stratification<br>- Indian caste system—origin and characteristics<br>- Positive and negative impact of caste in society<br>- Class system and status<br>- Social mobility—meaning and types<br>- Race—concept, criteria of racial classification<br>- Influence of class, caste and race system on health. | - Lecture<br>- Panel discussion | - Essay<br>- Short answer<br>- Objective type |
| VI | 15 (T) | Explain social organization, disorganization, social problems and role of nurse in reducing social problems | **Social organization and disorganization**<br>- Social organization—meaning, elements and types<br>- Voluntary associations<br>- Social system—definition, types, role and status as structural element of social system<br>- Interrelationship of institutions<br>- Social control—meaning, aims and process of social control | - Lecture<br>- Group discussion<br>- Observational visit | - Essay<br>- Short answer<br>- Objective type<br>- Visit report |

Contd...

*Contd...*

| Unit | Time (Hrs) | Learning Outcomes | Content | Teaching/Learning Activities | Assessment Methods |
|---|---|---|---|---|---|
| | | | <ul><li>Social norms, moral and values</li><li>Social disorganization—definition, causes, control and planning</li><li>Major social problems—poverty, housing, food supplies, illiteracy, prostitution, dowry, child labor, child abuse, delinquency, crime, substance abuse, HIV/AIDS, COVID-19</li><li>Vulnerable group—elderly, handicapped, minority and other marginal group</li><li>Fundamental rights of individual, women and children</li><li>Role of nurse in reducing social problem and enhance coping</li><li>Social welfare programs in India</li></ul> | | |
| VII | 5 (T) | Explain clinical sociology and its application in the hospital and community | **Clinical sociology**<ul><li>Introduction to clinical sociology</li><li>Sociological strategies for developing services for the abused</li><li>Use of clinical sociology in crisis intervention</li></ul> | <ul><li>Lecture</li><li>Group discussion</li><li>Role play</li></ul> | <ul><li>Essay</li><li>Short answer</li></ul> |

INC Syllabus  XIX

# CHAPTER 1

# An Introduction to Sociology

**Introduction**
- Meaning and definition
- Nature and scope of sociology
- Sociology and other social sciences
- Its relation to anthropology, psychology, social psychology, medical sociology
- Methods of social investigations
- Case study method
- Social survey method
- Questionnaire and interview method
- Opinion poll method
- Importance of its study with special reference to health care professionals

**Social factors in health and disease situations**

## ■ INTRODUCTION

Sociology is a social science. Medicine and social sciences are related. Social Medicine is a new speciality, which studies man as a social being in his total environment. The social sciences like Sociology, Psychology and Anthropology study man not only as a biological being but also as a social and cultural being. Social and economic factors have an influence on the health of the individual. Health and disease have social causes, social consequences and social therapies. Therefore, Prof. FAE Crew stated that social medicine stands on two pillars-Medicine and Sociology. Social Medicine is a new orientation of medicine to the changing needs of man and society. Health care professionals, as well as the social sciences are concerned with the human behavior. The health care professionals are seeking the help of social scientists in understanding the problems, such as the social component of health, disease and illness behavior of people.

Today, it is realized that man is a social animal and therefore, his health is affected by a number of factors other than his biological disposition like social, economic, educational status, cultural and behavioral factors. Social Sciences study man and society, the life and activities of man. They refer to the application of the scientific method to the study of intricate and complex network of human relationships and forms of organizations, desired to enable people to live together in societies. Social Sciences deal with the forms and contents of man's interactions. For example, History, Economics, Sociology, Psychology, Social Psychology, Social Anthropology and Political Science. They study the social conditions in which man lives. Social Sciences help in understanding and controlling social interactions. They are important in promoting human welfare. The whole of mankind and society is the laboratory for the social scientist.

The term "Behavioral Science" is applied to Sociology, Social Psychology and Social Anthropology because they deal with human behavior. "Man is a social animal". This was the statement made by the great Greek philosopher, Aristotle. It means that man cannot live alone. He has to have relationships or interactions with other men. These relationships give rise to behavior patterns and groups. Man has these relationships in order to survive. The study of all these phenomenons makes up "Sociology". The term sociology was first used by Auguste Comte (1798-1857), a French Philosopher, to describe these social phenomenon. Earlier all this was studied as a part of Philosophy.

The term "Sociology" is derived from the Latin word "societus" meaning "society" and the Greek word "logos" meaning "science" or "study". Therefore, the etymological meaning of the word "Sociology" is "the science or study of society". The term "society" again is a very broad one, which includes a number of aspects like man, his relationships, groups that he forms, his behavior patterns and so on. The subject matter of Sociology includes all this. Man is described not only as a social animal but also as a cultural and rational animal, which differentiates him from other animals in the society and places him higher than the other animals. The study of cultures of society also is an important part of Sociology.

History of society can be traced back to history of man and beginning of civilizations, when man had to live with his fellow beings and when he had to face problems and difficulties of living together. He had to naturally find solutions to his daily living. The systematic study of society began in the West in the early 19th century. Auguste Comte, a French Philosopher and Sociologist coined the term "Sociology" for the study of society. He defined Sociology as "a science of social phenomenon, subject to natural invariable laws, the discovery of which is the object of investigation". He advocated the use of positive method for sociological investigations in his work "Positive Philosophy". He is therefore known as the "Father of Sociology". Along with him other social thinkers like Herbert Spencer, Emile Durkheim, Karl Marx and Max Weber, also contributed to making of Sociology as a science. Therefore, these five thinkers are called as pioneers or founding fathers of Sociology. In the later half of 19th century and early 20th century, Sociology developed rapidly with contributions of a large number of Sociologists and social thinkers. Sociology also developed in India as an academic discipline after World War I. Some of prominent Sociologists of India are DP Mukherjee, GS Gharge. RK Mukerjee, Humanyan Kabir, KM Kapadia, RK Saxena, Mrs Iravati Karve, DN Mujamdar, MN Srinivas, MS Gore, SC Dube, PS Prabhu, AR Desai and others. The main aim of Sociology therefore, is to understand and acquire knowledge about the society.

## ■ DEFINITION

Sociology has been defined by different Sociologists in different ways each one taking different aspects of society for their definition. It is very difficult to give a single definition of Sociology, which would include all these aspects of the society and therefore, no single definition has been arrived at by them. For the purpose of study we may take up some of the important definitions.

Auguste Comte, the Father of Sociology, defines Sociology as "a science of social phenomena, subject to natural invariable laws, the discovery of which is the object of investigation".

Emile Durkheim defines Sociology as "the science of social institutions".

Max Weber defines Sociology as "the science which attempts the interpretative understanding of social actions".

HM Johnson defines it as "the science that deals with social groups, their internal forms or modes of organization, the processes that tend to maintain or change these forms of organization and relations between groups".

According to Kimbal and Young, it is "the science that deals with behavior of men in groups".

Mac Iver defines Sociology as "the science that seeks to discover the principles of cohesion and of order within social structure".

K Davis says that "Sociology is a general science of society".

Ogburn and Nimkoff defines it as "the scientific study of social life".

According to Henry Fairchild "it is the study of man and his environment".

Morris Ginsberg defines Sociology as "the study of human interactions and interrelations, their conditions and consequences".

From all these definitions cited above, it can be said that Sociology is a science of society, which attempts to study the social relationships of man, which is the basis of social interactions or social processes. While trying to understand these processes, the sociologists attempt to understand the evolution of society, its systems and structures development of social institutions and their functions, the social norms regulating the social relationships and social behavior and nature and interdependence of these groups, causes and consequences of changes in institutions and social organizations i.e. the phenomenon of social change.

## ■ NATURE OF SOCIOLOGY

Sociology is the study of sociely. Sciences are classified as pure or natural sciences and social sciences. The pure sciences like Physics, Chemistry, Mathematics, etc. deal with inanimate objects. These are more accurate and exact. On the other hand, the social sciences like History, Economics, Political Sciences, Sociology, Psychology, Anthropology, etc. deal broadly with man and society. All social sciences are interrelated and interdependent.

Sociology being a social science, studies man and society, the life and activities of man in the society. Social sciences refer to "the application of the scientific method to the study of intricate and complex network of human relationships and forms of organization desired to enable people to live together in the societies". Subjects like History, Economics, Political Sciences, Sociology, Anthropology, etc. deal with the forms and contents of man's interactions and the social conditions in which man lives. They help in understanding and controlling interactions. In addition, they are important in promoting human welfare. The whole of mankind and society is the laboratory for the social scientist.

## Sociology as a Science

Sociology has been defined as a "Science" more precisely as a "Social Science". What is Science? A Science may be defined as a method of study, a body of organized, verified knowledge, secured through scientific investigations. In this sense, Sociology therefore is a science because it has developed a body of organized, verified knowledge, which is based on scientific investigations and uses scientific methods of study. Sociology as a Science has its own distinctive characteristics, which distinguishes it from other sciences.

An understanding of these characteristics will help us to understand what kind of science it is. Some of the important characteristics of Sociology have been mentioned by Robert Biersted in his book "The Social Order".

1. Sociology is an independent science, which has its own field and method of study.
2. Sociology is a social science and not a physical or natural science. It studies man, his relationships, his behavior and groups that he forms. It is thus closely related and dependent upon other social sciences like History, Political Science, Economics, Anthropology, etc. and it can be distinguished from the natural sciences like Physics, Chemistry, Mathematics, etc.
3. Sociology is a categorical and not a normative discipline. Sociology studies "what is" and not "what should be or ought to be". It is ethically neutral i.e., it does not make any value judgments. This means that Sociology as a science cannot deal with problems of good and evil, right and wrong and moral or immoral.
4. Sociology is a pure or theoretical science. The aim is to acquire knowledge about the society. It has its own applied field. Each pure science has its own applied field. Sociology as a pure science is applied in the field of administration, social work, legislation, diplomacy, teaching, etc.
5. Sociology is relatively an abstract science and not a concrete science. It sociology studies man and the human events. It is concerned

with the form of human events and their patterns. It studies the social phenomena to these human events.
6. Sociology is a generalizing and not a particularizing or individualizing science. Sociology studies human events, which are innumerable. All of them cannot be studied. Therefore, it tries to make generalizations on the basis of some selected events.
7. Sociology is a general and not a special social science. It is the study of man and society as a whole, whereas other social sciences study only certain aspects of man and society.
8. Sociology is a rational and an empirical science. Any scientific knowledge can be gained through rational and empirical ways. Rational way stresses reasons and theories that result from logical inferences whereas empirical method is dependent on experience and facts that result from observation and experiment. Most sciences use both these methods for their studies. Sociology also is dependent on the rational, as well as the empirical method for its study.

Thus, from a study of these characteristics, it can be said that Sociology is an independent, categorical, pure, abstract, generalizing and a general social science, which uses both the rational and the empirical approach to gain scientific knowledge.

## ■ SCOPE OF SOCIOLOGY

Sociology has been defined as the science of man and society. It is the scientific study of human social life. Human beings have interactions and interrelations, which give rise to different kinds of groups. These groups have their own customs and traditions, develop their own institutions and create values. The group living in turn, is effected by these customs, traditions and values. It is interested in the way groups interact with one another and in the processes and institutions that they develop. Thus, it has a number of specialized fields like Sociology of Knowledge, Sociology of Religion, Sociology of Family and Marriage, Industrial Sociology, Rural Sociology, Urban Sociology, Medical Sociology, Health Sociology, Hospital Sociology, etc. The field of Sociology is thus very wide and covers almost every aspect of man and society

There are two main schools of thought regarding the scope of Sociology.

1. Specialistic or Formalistic School.
2. Synthetic School

## Specialistic or Formalistic School

Specialistic or Formalistic School was advocated by the German Sociologist Simmel and then followed by others like Small, Vierkandt, Max Weber, Von Wiese and Tonnies. According to them, Sociology studies one specific aspect of social relationships, i.e., forms in their abstract nature and not in any concrete situation. The form of social relationships do not change with a change in content of relationships. Thus, this school has limited the scope of Sociology to the abstract study of forms of social relationships.

## Synthetic School

Synthetic School of thought was advocated by Durkheim, Hobhouse, Sorokin, Karl Marx and Ginsberg. According to them, all parts of social life are intimately interrelated. The study of one aspect is not enough to understand the whole phenomenon. Sociology therefore, has to study social life as a whole.

Thus, it can be said that the scope of Sociology is very wide. It is a general, as well as a special science. The subject matter of all social sciences is society, but their view points are different. For example, Economics studies society from the economic point of view, Political Science from the political point of view, and History from the historical point of view. Sociology alone studies society as a whole. It studies all aspects of society like social groups, social processes, social structures, social institutions, social traditions, social systems, social stratifications, social changes, social pathologies, etc. It is neither possible nor essential to delimit the scope of Sociology.

## ■ SOCIOLOGY AND OTHER SOCIAL SCIENCES

Today, it is realized that man is a social animal and therefore his health is effected by a number of factors other than his biological disposition, like social, economic, educational status, cultural and behavioral factors.

Health care and social sciences are concerned with human behavior. Social sciences study man and society, the life and activities of man. They refer to "the application of the scientific method to the study of intricate and complex network of human relationships and forms of organizations desired to enable people to live together in societies. Social sciences deal with the forms and contents of man's interactions. For example, History, Economics, Sociology, Psychology, Social Psychology, Social Anthropology and Political Science. They study the social conditions in which man lives. Social sciences help in understanding and controlling social interactions. They are important in promoting human welfare. The whole of mankind and society is the laboratory for the social scientist. The term "behavioral science" is applied to Sociology, Social Psychology and Social Anthropology because they deal with human behavior.

## Sociology and Social Psychology

Sociology and Psychology are very closely related to each other. Sociology is the science of society, which attempts to study the social relationships of man, which is the basis of social interactions or social processes. Psychology is the study of human behavior. It is primarily concerned with the individual. It is the study of the mental processes of man. Social Psychology serves as a bridge between Sociology and Psychology. It deals with the mental processes of man, who is considered as a social being. Social psychology studies the characters of his social behavior like social interaction between an individual and a group and interaction between one group of individuals and another group of individuals. It studies the individual in relation to his fellow beings. Social psychology also studies how an individual's personality is dependent on social, cultural, physiological and temperamental factors.

### Differences between Sociology and Social Psychology

| Sociology | Social Psychology |
|---|---|
| Sociology is the study of the society as a whole. | Social Psychology is the study of the individual's behavior-his interaction as a group member. |

*Contd...*

*Contd...*

| Sociology | Social Psychology |
|---|---|
| Focus is on the society. | Focus is on the individual. |
| Analysis social processes. | Analysis mental processes. |
| Studies social forms and structures within which man behaves. | Primarily concerned with the study of man as such. |
| Studies the social groups and social structures within which the individual and group processes occur. | Studies the individual in the social groups. |
| Studies society from sociological point of view. | Studies individual from the psychological point of view. |

## Sociology and Anthropology

Anthropology is derived from the Greek words "Anthropos" meaning "man" and "logos" meaning "study" or "science". Thus, the etymological meaning of Anthropology is the scientific study of man as such, i.e. the study of the development of human race. Sociology and Anthropology have a very close relationship with each other. In fact anthropologist Kroeber pointed out that these two sciences are like twin sisters. Anthropology has a very wide field of study. It can be studied as

   i. Physical Anthropology which deals with the study of human evolution, racial differences, inheritance of bodily traits, growth and decay of the human organism.
   ii. Social Anthropology is the study of the development and various types of social life.
   iii. Cultural Anthropology is the study of the total way of life of man, his ways of thinking, feeling and action.

### Differences between Sociology and Anthropology

| Sociology | Anthropology |
|---|---|
| Studies modern civilized and complex societies, the social problems and suggest solutions. | Studies simple ancient communities and the problems existing therein. |
| Studies various aspects and problems of the society and guides for change like family, marriage, social processes, social change, and social mobility. | Studies societies as a whole. |

*Contd...*

*Contd...*

| Sociology | Anthropology |
|---|---|
| Studies social relationships of man. | Studies anatomical characteristics of man. |
| Makes suggestions for the future. | Tries to understand the past. |
| Makes use of documents, surveys, etc. for its study. | Uses the direct observation method for its study. |

## Sociology and Medical Sociology

### Medical Sociology

The field of Sociology extended towards medical science is known as "Medical Sociology". It is a specialization within the field of Sociology. Its main interest is health, health behavior and medical institutions. It includes studies of the medical profession, of the relationship of medicine to the public and of the social factors in the etiology, prevalence, incidence and interpretation of disease. Illness is viewed not only as a medical problem but also as a socio-psychological problem. The problems of the patients are not always medical. Diseases like tuberculosis, leprosy, sexually transmitted diseases, have a social component. Therefore, a social approach to disease treatment is emphasized.

Health is related to the social context. The social and economic factors have an influence on the health of the individual. They have an influence on the incidences, course and outcome of communicable disease, non-communicable diseases and many other health problems. The social and economic factors also have an effect on the provision of health care to the people in the society. Poverty, malnutrition, poor sanitation, lack of education, inadequate housing, unemployment, poor working conditions, cultural and behavioral factors, influence the health of the individuals. Man is considered as a social animal with personal idiosyncrasies, erratic habits, customs and beliefs, reacting on his body and mind. Thus, concepts of Sociology are increasingly being used in the study of health in human societies.

Medicine and social sciences are concerned in their own way with human behavior specially community health, clinical medicines and epidemiology, are all dependent on social sciences in understanding the problems, such as the social component of health and disease, "illness behavior" of people, efficient use of medical care and the study of medical institutions.

## Medical Sociology and Social Medicine

The field of Sociology, which is extended towards medical sciences is known as Medical Sociology. It describes medicine as a social science. There is a need to integrate the behavioral sciences with medicine in the education of health care professionals. Education, medicine, health care and socio-behavioral sciences are included in social medicine. The health care professionals would thus get a better understanding of the society. It studies the relationships between health factors and sociocultural, economic and political factors and the health behavior of the people.

Social medicine originated in Europe in the late 19th century. It stresses the importance of social factors in etiology of diseases. development in the field of social sciences like sociology, psychology and others showed that man is not only a biological animal but also social animal. Diseases have social causes, social consequences and social therapy. Thus, social medicine is a study of man as a social being in his total environment it focuses on the health of the community as a whole it gives importance to social factors as determinants of health and disease, it is concerned with all factors effecting health and ill-health of the population, including the use of health services. It shows the relationship between medicine and social sciences.

### *Social Telesis*

Social telesis is a planned progress and purposeful use of natural and social forces. It is a total process of cultural transformation. It is an indication for the quality of life, social change, social development and social control. e.g., in satellite programs, adult education, free education, etc. Bogardus describes social telesis as a process used for economic development, regional and rural development.

### *Medical Social Work*

Medical social work is an important field of social work and an integral part of medicine. It uses "case work" as a technique to find out the social background of illness. It helps the health care professional in arriving at a social diagnosis for treating the illness and arriving at a prognosis. The purpose is to help the sick people, both through the best use of patients' capabilities and the community resources in matters of personal and social adjustments in the community, including rehabilitation. The best person to do this kind of work is one who is specially trained in social case work i.e. the medical social worker.

### Medical Social Worker

The medical social worker is a paramedical worker, who has been trained in social case work and in interviewing people. They are employed in medical and public health organizations like hospitals, tuberculosis clinics, family planning clinics, cancer control centers, mental health centers, maternal and child welfare centers, and school and university health centers. The medical social worker is a link between the institution and the community. His main work is to visit the family and find out the personal economic and social causes of illness and collect the social history of the patient to supplement the medical history. He also tries to get help to the patient through community resources. In addition, the medical social worker helps in the rehabilitation of patients with chronic illnesses like leprosy, tuberculosis and polio. He is recognized as an important professional colleague of the medical practitioner.

## ■ METHODS OF SOCIAL INVESTIGATIONS

### Social Survey Method

Social survey method is one of the most important techniques of research in social sciences. It is a way of seeking social facts. It is concerned with the collection of data, relating to some social problems and formulating a constructive program for its solution. It is conducted within a fixed geographical area. Some of the main forms of social surveys are:
    i. General or specialized surveys.
    ii. Census or sample surveys.
    iii. Direct or indirect surveys.

iv. Official, semi-official or private surveys.
v. Wide spread or limited surveys.
vi. Public or confidential surveys.
vii. Initial or repetitive surveys.
viii. Primary or secondary surveys.
ix. Postal or personal surveys.
x. Regular or ad hoc surveys.

The social survey method is useful to obtain demographic data, information about people's behavior like their attitudes, opinions and interests. Thus, it helps to provide social and economic facts about the people in a particular area. This data may be useful to the government to understand and solve the social problems in a particular area. Social surveys may depend on the questionnaires, which are self-administered, schedules, which are completed by trained interviewers or by a research worker personally.

## Case-Study Method

Case-study method is an intensive investigation of a social unit. It is a form of qualitative analysis involving very careful observation of a person, a situation or an institution. It analyzes a limited number of events or conditions and their interrelations. The unit is taken as a representative of the group. Some of the sources of case study are personal documents like dieters, autobiography, memoirs, letters, etc. and life history. The data is collected through observation, interviews, questionnaires, government, voluntary or private agencies, co-opinionaires, psychological tests, and inventories and recorded data. This method is used in child care and child guidance institutions, schools, colleges, medical and psychiatric settings, family welfare and marriage counseling centers, institutions for the old and infirm, as well as handicapped and also with people who suffer from addiction, character disorders, emotional disturbances and the like.

## Questionnaire and Interview Method

Questionnaire and interview methods have become a very common form of data collection in sociological research. Questionnaire is useful for collecting data from a large number of people spread over a large area, especially about a particular situation or problem like personal preferences, social beliefs, attitudes, opinions, behavior patterns, group practices, habits etc.

### Questionnaire Method

Questionnaire consists of a set of questions, printed or typed, sent to the respondents, personally or through mail. It may be a structured questionnaire or an unstructured questionnaire.

i. Structured questionnaires are those, which have definite, concrete and prepared questions.
   They may be of
   a. Closed form type, where there are a number of alternative answers, given at the end of each question and respondent has to choose one of them. It is also called as the poll-type or selective-type questionnaire.
   b. Open-end type, where there are no readymade answers for the questions asked. The respondent is free to think and answer on his own. This is also called the inventive type, for the respondent has to think or invent the answers. Structured questionnaires are used in the study of socioeconomic problems, measurement of public-opinion, administrative policies, studies on consumer expenditure, cost of living, child welfare, public health and other issues.

ii. Unstructured questionnaires contain definite subject matter. It is precise and flexible. It is used to get views, opinions, attitudes, etc. There are no limitations and no predetermined responses provided. It is used for detailed studies like family group cohesiveness, studies of personal experiences, beliefs and attitudes.

### Interview Method

Interview method is an oral method. It is an important method of collecting data in social research. In this method, one person asks questions to another person, either in person, directly or indirectly, for a specific purpose. It is an effective information, verbal or non-verbal conversation. In general, interview method is a face-to-face verbal exchange of information or expressions of opinion from one person to another, regarding a particular issue. Some of the important types of interview are clinical interview, selection interview, diagnostic interview, research interview, directive interview, non-directive interview, focused or controlled interview, repeated interview, respondent interview and depth interview.

## Opinion Poll Method

Opinion poll method is used to collect data about a specific social phenomenon from a huge sample at a given time, spread over a large area. For example, this method is used to get information about the beliefs, attitudes, sentiments of the public on any given proposition like social, economic and political situations. The results of such public polls help the authorities concerned to modify their policies accordingly.

## ■ IMPORTANCE OF SOCIOLOGY

Sociology has been defined as the science of society and social phenomenon. The study of Sociology therefore, gives us a proper and better understanding and knowledge of the society. Its study is therefore important and has a great value for us.

1. Sociology is the scientific study of society. Before the emergence of Sociology, there was no scientific study of society or social phenomenon. They were studied as part of other social sciences. This scientific knowledge about society is required to achieve improvement and progress in different fields.
2. Sociology studies the role of institutions like marriage and family, school and education, state and government, industry and work, and church and religion, in the life of individuals, through which the society functions. They condition the individual's life. The knowledge of Sociology helps to strengthen them to serve man better.
3. Sociological knowledge is helpful for understanding and planning of the society. Social planning and social policies become effective with a knowledge of Sociology. It plays an important role in social reforms and reorganization.
4. Sociological knowledge is helpful for solving social problems. It helps in solving many social problems existing in today's modern world like over-population, unemployment, poverty, family and community disorganization, crime, juvenile delinquency, etc.

Sociology studies these problems through scientific methods and tries to find solutions to them.

5. Sociology has drawn our attention to the intrinsic worth and dignity of man. It has changed the ideas and attitudes of man towards fellow human beings. Sociology has made them broad minded. Factors like caste, creed, race, color and others, which created differences among men, are gradually loosing their importance for man.
6. Sociology has changed man's outlook with regard to problems of crime and juvenile delinquency. The criminals are treated as human beings suffering from some mental deficiencies. Knowledge of Sociology gives us a better understanding of the problems of crime and juvenile delinquency. Remedial measures are taken to rehabilitate them and make them normal members of the society.
7. Sociology makes a scientific study of cultures. Culture is a way of life of the people. They differ from people to people and place to place. Sociology helps man in taking a rational approach towards important aspects of culture like religion, customs, traditions, beliefs, ideas, values and ideals, attitudes, etc. It has made a great contribution to enrich human culture.
8. Sociology is useful as a teaching subject and is becoming an important teaching subject. It has an important place in the curriculum of colleges and universities. It is also included as a subject for competitive examinations like the Indian Administrative Services (IAS).
9. The study of Sociology is helpful for a number of professions. It will help students to get jobs as labour-welfare officers, human-relations officers, personnel officers in government offices and factories, in employment exchanges and social security schemes etc. as probationary officers, youth-welfare officers, rural-welfare officers, child-welfare officers, tribal-welfare officers, social-education officers, adult-education officers, widow-welfare officers, welfare-officers in homes established for old, disabled, destitutes, as a social worker or research student.
10. Sociology helps us to study and understand social phenomenon and of means and ways of promoting "Social adequacy" i.e. social welfare. As Prof. Giddings points out. "Sociology tells us

how to become what we want to be". The knowledge of Sociology has both individual and social advantages.

## Uses of Sociology in Nursing and Health Care Professions

The study of Sociology has been added recently in the study of Medical Education. The knowledge of Sociology is required for all Medical professions like Nursing, Physiotherapy and other health care professions because social factors and conditions play an important role in the health of the individual and society. Sociology will give them a knowledge of these factors and conditions, which will help them to give a proper treatment.

1. Nurses play an important role in health care. They work for healthier life style and better standards of living because they can influence the individuals in the society.
2. Nurses have to work in co-ordination with a number of institutions in the society like family, state, religion, governmental agencies and others, to implement health care activities.
3. Nurses have to provide love and care to patients that they come across in the hospitals or in the community. They can there by understand and meet the needs of the individual and the family.
4. Sociology will help to broaden the views of nurses. They will be able to understand human behavior and problems of the patients, which will help them to have a better interaction with their patients.
5. Knowledge of Sociology will help nurses to provide health counseling to patients, families, community agencies and groups of persons.
6. Sociology will help nurses to provide right motivation, treatment (physical, medical, vocational, psycho-social rehabilitation) based on attitudes and responses of patients by understanding their behavior through good interpersonal relationships.
7. Sociology will help the nurse to understand the emotional reactions of the people around her.
8. Sociology will help the nurse to understand the problems of patients because of her having a close and continuous contact with them in relation to their illness and disease.

9. Knowledge of Sociology helps the nurse to have a good observation, communication and guidance skills to understand patient's behavior.
10. Nurses have the responsibility for the provision of care in the community. They act as agents of social change to bring about good quality of life for the people. It helps them to have good relationship with the people.
11. It makes them sensitive to the health needs of the people in the context of broader social change.
12. The role of the nurse is that of an educator for health for all. Nurse has to take up health education activities in the community for which knowledge of Sociology is helpful.
13. Nurse has to act as a community organizer and leader in planning, organizing and implementing health services through the community participation.
14. Knowledge of Sociology will help the nurse to understand and make a diagnosis of sociocultural barriers like peoples beliefs, practices, customs, values, attitudes, traditions, to diseases, course of treatment, prevention of diseases and promotion of health. This will help the nurse to develop a plan of operation by involving the people and to have cultural perception and cultural meaning of health problems.
15. Nurses have to work with a number of people in the hospital situation like the doctor, the supervisor, subordinates, patients and their relations, visitors and others. It will help them to establish good social interactions and social relations with all of them.
16. The social problems affecting patients can be understood in a better way with a knowledge of Sociology. Remedies can be suggested to either solve them or to have a proper approach towards them.
17. It will help the nurse to identify and analyze different social situations, which give rise to conditions of diseases, epidemics, morbidity, mortality, etc. Knowledge of sociology will help in clinical practice and clinical teaching.

The role of the nurse is very important in health care services like preventive, promotive, curative, rehabilitative and restorative, which will bring her close to the people, thus acting as an agent of change in bringing a good quality of life to the people. Nurses will act as direct health care providers in meeting the health needs of the community. They should motivate the community to actively participate and involve in planning and implementing health care programs for attaining a good quality of life by selecting proper health education methods.

## ■ SOCIAL FACTORS IN HEALTH AND DISEASE SITUATIONS

1. Meaning of social factors.
2. Role of social factors in health and illness.

The concepts of health, disease and illness are all closely related to each other. It is important to understand these concepts for all health care professionals. Today, health is recognized as a fundamental human right. It is required for the satisfaction of the basic human needs and to improve the quality of life of the individuals. Health is a major instrument of over-all socio-economic development. It has been realized that it is not only a bio-medical concept, but one which is influenced by social, economic and political factors. Thus, it is both a biological and a social phenomenon.

The definition of health given by the World Health Organization (WHO) is as follows:

"Health is a state of complete physical, mental and social well being and not merely an absence of disease or infirmity". Social well-being of the individual is influenced by the world in which he lives. The social dimension of health includes the social functioning and ability to see oneself as a member of the larger society. Social health implies that every individual is a part of the family, the community and focuses on the social and economic conditions and well-being of the total individual in the context of his social relationships. Health is influenced by a number of factors, which lie both within the individual and externally in the society in which he lives.

Some of the important social factors that influence the health status of the people in the society are the following:

Behavioral and socio-cultural conditions have an influence on health. "Lifestyle" is one of the important determinants of health and disease. The term "lifestyle" is used to denote "the way people live". It includes their social values, attitudes and activities. Lifestyle includes the cultural and behavioral patterns and personal habits like smoking or alcoholism, which develop through the process of socialization. These lifestyles are learnt through interaction with parents, peer-groups, schools, siblings, and mass media. Therefore, a good health requires a good and healthy lifestyle.

Health and lifestyle of the people are related. Many health problems, especially in developed countries can be related to lifestyle like heart-disease, obesity, cancer, addiction, etc. But, in developing countries like India, where the traditional lifestyles still persists, risks of illness and death are related to a lack of sanitation, poor nutrition, personal hygiene, elementary human habits, customs and cultural patterns. It must be noted that not all lifestyle patterns are bad for health. Some lifestyle factors are good for maintaining the health of the population like good nutrition, enough sleep, sufficient physical activity, etc.

Socioeconomic conditions influence human health. Health is dependent upon the social and economic development of the society like the per capita income, G.N.P, education, nutrition, employment, housing, political system of the country, etc.

Health and family welfare services also play an important role in the treatment of disease, prevention of illness and promotion of health. Health services are necessary for maintaining and improving the health of the population and for the social and economic development of the society. There is a dependency of health on socio-economic factors like health services, literacy levels, unemployment, adequate housing facilities, sanitation and food, which results in a poor quality of life.

The concept of disease is related to the concept of health. According to the Oxford English Dictionary, disease is "a condition of the body or some part or organ of the body in which its functions are disrupted or deranged." From a sociological point of view, disease is a social phenomenon occurring in all societies. In general, it can be said that it is any deviation from the normal functioning or a state of complete physical or mental well-being.

A number of factors are responsible for a disease condition. Psychosocial factors are those factors, which take into consideration the fact that man is a social psychological and cultural being. Therefore, these factors effect his personal health, health care and community well-being. They include cultural values, customs, habits, beliefs, attitudes, morals, religion, education, lifestyles, community life, health services social and political organization.

Man being a social animal is in constant interaction with people around him. He is a member of a social group, a family, a caste, a community, a nation and so on. Therefore, one man's behavior effects another man. The social controls like laws, customs, traditions, attitudes, beliefs, values etc., regulate their interrelationships. This is the social environment, which has both positive and negative impact on the health of the individual and the communities. A good social environment can improve the health of the individual and improve the quality of life also. Therefore, good customs and traditions favoring health must be preserved. Some psychosocial factors also have a negative effect on man's health and well-being like poverty, urbanization and industrialization, accompanied by migration and stressful situations, may produce feelings of anxiety, depression, anger, frustration, and so on, which may lead to some physical symptoms, such as headache, palpitations and sweating. These emotional changes also produce structural changes in various organs of the body, resulting in psychosomatic disorders like duodenal ulcer, bronchial asthma, hypertension, heart diseases, mental disorders and deviant behaviors like crime, suicide, violence, drug abuse, alcoholism, etc. From a psychosocial point of view a disease may be viewed as maladjustment of the human organism to his psychosocial environment. For example, smoking as a behavior and habit can be considered as a psychosocial cause for certain diseases like lung cancer.

Rehabilitation medicine is another medical specialty in recent times. It involves disciplines, such as physical medicine or physiotherapy, occupational therapy, speech therapy, audiology, psychology, education, social work, vocational guidance and placement services. Rehabilitation medicine helps the individuals to achieve social integration and become normal human beings, actively participating in the community life. Rehabilitation has been defined as "the combined and coordinated use of medical, social,

educational and vocational measures for training and retraining the individuals to the highest possible level of functional ability." The following are the types of rehabilitation:
1. Medical rehabilitation – restoration of function.
2. Vocational rehabilitation – restoration of the capacity to earn a living.
3. Social rehabilitation – restoration of family and social relationships.
4. Psychological rehabilitation – restoration of personal dignity and confidence.

All these different types of rehabilitations have to be used by the health care professionals to bring back their disabled, handicapped and the diseased patients to normalcy.

From the above discussion it is clear that there is a relationship of Sociology with the health sciences. The study of Sociology helps the health care professional to understand the patient's social environment, which is very essential in the treatment of any health problem. Sociological knowledge can also be applied in the prevention and treatment of illness and in rehabilitating the patients. Thus, we understand the patient in his social context and to rehabilitate him in all aspects, the study of Sociology is essential for all health care professionals.

### POINTS TO NOTE
1. Definition–meaning–scope of sociology.
2. Importance of the study especially for health care professional.
3. Relationship with other social sciences like anthropology–psychology–social psychology–medical sociology.
4. Methods of social investigations–case study method–social survey method–questionnaire and interview method–opinion poll method.
5. Social factors in health and disease conditions.

### NURSING IMPLICATIONS
Importance of the study of sociology for health care professionals to understand the patient's social environment for the treatment of the health disease, prevention and treatment of illness and in rehabilitation of patients.

## QUESTIONS

1. Define the following:
   a. Sociology
   b. Science
   c. Social Science
   d. Medico social science
   e. Social Telesis
   f. Medical social worker
   g. Medical sociology
2. "Man is a social animal" – Discuss.
3. Explain the role of nurses in society.
4. Bring out the social factors influencing health and illness.
5. Define Sociology. Explain the importance of the study of Sociology.
6. Write the meaning of the root words from which Sociology is derived.
7. Describe the origin and developments of Social Medicine. What is its application in nursing?
8. Describe the sociological research methods used in health care profession.
9. Define Sociology. Discuss the importance of the study of Sociology in nursing.
   Or
   Write an essay on the significance of Sociology in the nursing profession.
10. Describe the nature and scope of Sociology. How does Sociology help in nursing profession?

# CHAPTER 2

# Man and Society

- Meaning-definition-factors-stages-agencies-types
- Nature of society
- Difference between society and community
- Process of socialization
- Individualization

"Man is a social animal". This was the statement that the great Greek Philosopher, Aristotle made thousands of years ago. It means that man cannot live alone. He needs the company of fellow human beings all through his life for his social, psychological and economic well-being.

Auguste Comte, the French Philosopher, coined the word "Sociology" from the two words "Societus" and "Logos". The word Societus" means "society" and thereby he defined Sociology as the "science of society". The word "society" is a very common word, used in our daily language to mean people coming together to form groups like the Theosophical Society or the Society for the Prevention of Cruelty to Animals or primitive society, civilized society or urban society or rural society or tribal society. But the meaning of the term as used in Sociology is different. In order to understand this term, we take up some of the definitions of society.

## ■ DEFINITION

1. Mac Iver and Page "Society is a system of usages and procedures, authority and mutual aid, of many groupings and divisions, of control of human behavior and of liberties" i.e., it is a "web of social relationships."
2. Prof. Wright "Society is not a group of people; it is a system of relationships that exist between individuals of groups."
3. Ginsberg "A society is a collection of individuals united by certain relations or modes of behavior, which mark them off from others

who do not enter into these relations or who differ from them in behavior."
4. T. Parsons "Society may be defined as the total complex of human relationships in so far as they grow out of action in terms of mean-end relationships, intrinsic or symbolic."
5. La Piere "The term society refers not to a group of people, but to a complex pattern of norms of interaction that arise among and between them."

From the above definitions, it is clear that society includes mutual interactions and mutual interrelations of individuals and it is a structure formed by these relations. It is thus a pattern, a system and not the people.

Thus, it can be said that "society" is defined from two points of view by sociologists.
1. From the functional point of view where it is understood as a complex of groups in reciprocal relationships interacting with one another in their daily activities.
2. From the structural point of view, society is a total social heritage of folkways, mores and institutions, of habits, sentiments and ideals.

Mac Iver defines society as "a web of social relationships." What is a social relationship then? All relationships of man cannot be defined as social. For example, if there are two people waiting at the bus stop for a bus, independent of each other, there is no social relationship between them. But, as soon as they become aware of each other, the element of sociality comes in. A social relationship therefore, implies reciprocal awareness between two or more people and the sense of their having something in common. Thus, reciprocal recognition and commonness are characteristic feature of every social relationship.

## Elements of Society

Mac Iver defines society as a system of usages and procedures, authority and mutual aid, of many groupings and divisions, of controls of human behavior and of liberties. From this definition, it follows that the elements of society are the following:
1. In every society, there are certain usages concerned with important aspects of life like marriage, education, religion, food, language, etc. These differ from society to society.

2. There are certain procedures i.e., ways of action in every society, which maintain its unity and organization.
3. The presence an authority to maintain its order.
4. Stability of the society is maintained by mutual aid among its members.
5. In every society there are a number of groups and divisions like family, tribe, village, town, city, etc.
6. Controls are essential for the organization of the society.
7. Liberty or freedom helps man to develop his personality and individuality.

## Characteristics of Society

1. Society is made up of people.
2. These people have a mutual awareness and mutual interaction, which gives rise to social relationships.
3. Society has likeness or similarities. There are similarities among people where their likes, needs, aims, ideals, values, outlook towards life, etc. are concerned.
4. Society also has differences. There are differences among people because they have varied interests. Also, they differ in their looks, personality, ability, talent, attitudes, interests, intelligence and so on. No two people are the same. These differences make life more interesting. Thus, there are differences in the society in all aspects of life. For example, people are engaged in different kinds of economic activities in the society like farmers, teachers, laborers, engineers, doctors, nurses, etc. for their survival.
5. There is cooperation and division of labor in society. Likeness and differences give rise to division of labor and cooperation. Division of labor is possible because of cooperation, which leads to a great amount of specialization, a characteristic of modern complex societies. Division of labor increases the interdependence, interrelations and interactions among the people and groups. Thus, it is based on cooperation. This results in social cohesion and social solidarity, by which people are able to satisfy their common needs, interests and desires.
6. Interdependence is required among the people, groups and communities to meet the societal needs.

Man and Society 27

7. Society is dynamic and not static. Changes keep occurring continuously in the society i.e., it is dynamic. Change may take place abruptly or slowly or gradually or suddenly.
8. There are a number of social processes like competition, conflicts, tensions, revolts, etc. which disturb the social order of the society. Society has its own ways and means of controlling the people's behavior and maintaining the social peace and order in the form of social controls. These social controls may be of the formal type like laws, police, courts, judges, army and others or the informal type like the customs traditions, folkways and others.
9. Every society has its own culture i.e., its own way of life, which makes it different from others. Culture and society go together. Culture is the learned behavior pattern of man and the groups that he forms. That is why, man is also called as a cultural being, which distinguishes him from the other animals in the society. It is the sum of what the group has learnt about living together. It is an important element of society.
10. Man is gregarious by nature. Man is a social animal i.e., he cannot live alone. He needs the company of others in order to develop his personality as a normal human being. Man can become man only in the company of other men i.e., man is gregarious by nature. Gregarious means the tendency of man to live in groups. This instinctive nature of man has forced him to establish social groups and societies and to live in them. Man and society go together. Man is born in the society. He is nourished and nurtured from his birth till his death in the society.

## ■ COMMUNITY AND ASSOCIATION

Community and association are the most important types of social groups. A community is a permanent social group, embracing a totality of ends or purposes. The members live their life in a community. Here they are able to find all their social relations. The interests and aims of individuals forming a community are fulfilled within it. In this sense it is a self-contained group. A community has its own structure and rules by which its members are governed and thus have a common way of life. It has a number of associations and institutions within its framework. The members thereby are able to satisfy their individual, as well as social interests. Also, a smaller community exists within a large community e.g., joint family in the Indian villages.

An association on the other hand is a group of people united for a specific purpose or a limited number of purposes. For example, an army for the defence of the nation or a school for imparting education. An association is thus a voluntary group formed with a certain purpose or aim and the members work together to achieve that end or aim. They exist within the community for fulfilling the interests of the individuals.

The term "community" like the term "society" is also used in our daily language. It is used by different people to mean different things. For example, religious community, linguistic community and minority community. But in Sociology, the term "community" is used to mean a social group. In order to understand the meaning of the term, we take up some important definitions.

## Definitions

1. *Bogardus*—A social group with a "we feeling" and "living in a given area".
2. *Mac Iver*—An area of social living marked by some degree of coherence.
3. *Kingsley Davis*—The smallest territorial group that can embrace all aspects of social life.
4. *Lundberg*—A human population living within a limited geographic area and carrying on a common interdependent life.
5. *Ogburn and Nimkoff*—The total organization of social life within a limited area.
6. *Manheim*—Any circle of people who live together and belong together in such a way that they do not share this or that particular interest only but a whole set of interests.

From the above definitions, it is clear that a community is a group of people living in a given geographical area and sharing a common way of life or a sense of belonging i.e., a "we feeling". Thus, it includes all our social relationships and a variety of associations and institutions like economic, political, religious, educational and other activities. The community is the total organization of social life within a given geographical area like a tribe, a village, a town, a city, etc.

## Elements or Characteristics of Community

Some of the important elements on the basis of which a group can be identified as a community are the following:
1. *Group of people*—Community is a group of people sharing the basic conditions of common life.
2. *Locality*—A group of people form a community, when they start living in a particular geographical area. Living together in a locality, a strong bond of solidarity develops among the people. They are able to develop and fulfill their common interests within community. The physical and natural conditions of the locality like the soil, water, vegetation, forests, climate, etc. influence the life of the people living there. These factors influence the economic activities of the community.
3. *Community sentiment*—When people start living in a geographical area, they start having a common feeling or a "we feeling" i.e., they start having a feeling of belonging together. This is called the community sentiment. Thus, in a community, there is a sense of identification, a sense of awareness, a sense of living and sharing some common interests in life.
4. *Permanency*—Community includes a permanent group of life. It is not temporary and therefore, it has stability.
5. *Naturality*—Community gets established naturally. It is not manmade. Man is born into it and thus becomes the member of a community.
6. *Likeness*—People in a community share a common way of life. They have a common language, customs, traditions, folkways, mores, etc., which regulate their behavior patterns.
7. *Wider ends*—The membership in a community is natural. People do not associate with it for any particular end. The ends of a community are much wider.
8. *Particular name*—Every community has a particular name, which indicates the identity, reality and individuality. Each community is something of a personality.
9. *Legal state*—Community has no legal status.
10. *Size of community*—Size of the community may be big or small. Smaller communities are included within a larger community. Hence, there are communities within communities.

**Differences between Society and Community**

| Society | Community |
|---|---|
| Society is a web of social relationships. | Community is a group of people living in a given geographical area and sharing a "we feeling". |
| Society is abstract. | Community is concrete. |
| It is not necessary to have a definite locality for a society. | A well-defined geographical area is necessary for a community. |
| Community sentiment as "we feeling" may or may not be present. | Community sentiment is an essential element of community. |
| Society is wider. It may include more than one community in it. | Community is smaller than society. It exists within the society. |
| Common objectives and interests of society are wider. | Community objectives and interests are comparatively less extensive and varied. |
| Society includes both likeness and difference. | Common agreement of interests and objectives are necessary in community. |

# ■ PROCESS OF SOCIALIZATION

## Concept and Meaning of Socialization

The human child comes into this world as a biological being with animal needs. He is gradually moulded into a social being by learning the social ways of acting and feeling from others in the society. Every society or social group has its own culture, i.e., its own way of life, with its own rules and practices for its members. These rules and practices, which are also called as norms of society or the set of standard behavior patterns of society, maintain the peace and order of the society. The individual, born into the group, learns these norms in the process of his growth from different people around him. This is the moulding of the personality of the individual. Without this process, the society would not be able to continue, nor the culture exist nor the individual become a personality. This process of moulding is called "socialization".

Socialization therefore, is a learning process. Man learns a set of attitudes, habits, skills, standards, values, likes, dislikes, goals and purposes, judgments and patterns of behavior that are necessary for the individuals effective participation in social groups and communities. This learning is a continuous process. It starts from the time of the birth of the individual and continues throughout his life and ends at the time of his death only. It is through this process that the individual internalizes the norms of the society. That is, the norms become a part of the individual's personality.

## Definitions

1. *Ogburn*—The process by which the individual learns to confirm to the group norms.
2. *Peter Worsley*—The process of transmission of culture, whereby the individuals learn the rules and practices of social groups.
3. *Harry M Johnson*—It enables the learner to perform social roles and transmit culture.
4. *Horton and Hunt*—One internalizes the norms of his groups so that a distinct "self" emerges, unique to that particular individual.
5. *Majumdar*—The process whereby the original nature is transformed into human nature and the individual into a person.

From the above definitions, it is clear that socialization is a continuous learning process in the life of the individual, beginning from the time of his birth and ending at his death. It maintains the social order and peace in the society by making man a good social and cultural being. It shapes the total personality of the individual. It is the most important factor in the development of the personality of the individual.

## Factors in the Process of Socialization

Socialization is the process of learning the group norms of the society. The important factors that help in this process of learning are the following:

1. *Imitation*—Imitation is the copying by an individual of acts or behavior patterns of another Individual. Child has the greatest capacity to imitate. The children have the greatest influence of their parents and others whose behavior they immediately pick-up. It may be spontaneous or deliberate, conscious or unconscious, perceptual or ideational. For example, the boys tend

to imitate the elder men, like their father in the family. Language and pronunciation are learnt by the child through imitation.
2. *Suggestion*—Suggestion is the process of communicating information, which has no logical or rational basis from one to another. It can be conveyed through language and several other mass media. Intellectual ability plays as important role in suggestion. Therefore, it is very easy to influence a child through suggestions as he is still not mature intellectually. Socialization of the child through this method becomes easy, whereas an adult cannot be very easily influenced by suggestions as he is mentally more mature.
3. *Identification*—In early childhood a child cannot make a distinction between his organism and environment. Most of his behavior and actions are random and unconscious. It is only with age, that he learns to identify things, which satisfy his needs. Such things become the objects of his identification.
4. *Language*—Language is the medium of communication and social interaction. It is a means of cultural transmission. At first, the child does not have any language. As it grows up, it learns a language from the others around it. It is through this medium of language that the child gets socialized by others around it and it helps him to develop his personality right from infancy.

## Stages of Socializations

Socializations is a process, which goes on gradually throughout the individual's life. It starts from infancy and goes on to adulthood. Socializations is a process that goes from a simple form to a more complex form in his growth and development in society. He learns the standard norms of society, which will help him to play the social roles and also to understand the social roles played by others, so that he is able to interact with them. At each stage of socialization, child internalizes a "system" of roles.

Socialization is carried on in four stages from infancy to adulthood. They are:
1. Oral stage.
2. Anal stage.
3. Oedipal stage.
4. Adolescence stage.

1. *The First Stage-The Oral stage*—This stage starts from birth and continues up to one year. In the womb, the child has a comfortable environment, completely protected. As he comes out, he has to face the first crisis i.e., he must breathe, exert himself to feed, must be protected from physical discomforts. The child gradually learns to give signals to satisfy its needs. This it does by crying. By crying, the child establishes its oral dependency. Sigmund Freud called this stage as "primary identification" i.e., the child merges his identity with that of the mother.
2. *The Second Stage-The Anal Stage*—This stage begins after the first year and is completed by the third year. In this stage, the mother tries to gradually wean away the child from her. She does this, by training him to become independent and take care of himself. He is taught to do some small tasks, such as toileting, wearing clothes, etc. "Toilet training" therefore becomes the main focus in this stage. The child learns about the two separate roles - his own role and that of his mother. He also learns to distinguish between right and wrong or correct and incorrect actions.
3. *The Third Stage-The Oedipal Stage*—This stage starts from the fourth year and goes on up to the twelfth or thirteenth year. The child starts identifying himself as a member of the family. He starts identifying himself with the social roles as ascribed to him on the basis of sex. According to Freud, the boy develops the "Oedipus complex" i.e., feeling of jealousy towards father and love towards the mother and the girl develops "Electra complex" i.e., feeling of jealousy towards the mother and love for the father. There is a great amount of social pressure on the child to identify himself with the right sex. The parents help the child to make the proper sex identification. About the age of six, the child is able to understand sexual differences. The boy generally identifies himself with the father and the girl with the mother. Thus, in this stage, the child internalizes his role, the role of the father, mother and other siblings.
4. *The Fourth Stage-Adolescence stage*—This stage starts with the onset of adolescence and continuous into adulthood. This is the stage between young age and adulthood. It is a period

of transition, when the individual experiences a number of physiological, as well as psychological changes. This stage therefore, has a great importance because the individual will be in a state of confusion and conflict within himself. During this stage, the individual likes to free himself from parental control, while still being dependent on his parents. He wants to have freedom in doing various things while the parents want to control many of his activities. This causes a lot of strain and conflict within him.

## ■ AGENCIES OF SOCIALIZATION

Socialization is the shaping or moulding of individuals, whereby individuals develop qualities essential for functioning effectively in the society in which they are living. It is a process, which begins at the time of birth of the individual and continues throughout his life, till his death. The child's socialization should not be left to mere accident but it should be controlled through institutional channels. The following are the agencies of socialization that have been established by culture.

1. *The Family and Parents*—The family is one of the most important primary groups in the society. The child is born into the family. It is here that the child learns the ways of life of the society into which he is born, through his parents. The parents, especially the mother, has a great role to play in the socialization of the child. They are not only closely related to him but they are physically very close to him. Therefore, they have a great influence on the moulding of the personality of the child. From the parents, he learns his speech and language, social values, cooperation, tolerance, self-sacrifice, love and affection. For example, in a bad family, the child learns bad habits, whereas in a good family he acquires good habits.
2. *The School and Teachers*—The school and teachers are the second important agency of socialization. It is a here that the child is given a formal education, which moulds his ideas and attitudes. Culture is formally transmitted and acquired from one generation to the next. This socialization makes them mature members of the society.
3. *Peer Group*—Peer group is the group of friends or playmates, generally of the same age. It is also called as the age mates. An

individual has his group of peers at every age during his lifetime and is continuously influenced by them. As he grows up, the peer group becomes more important for him than the parental group. The peer group exerts a great amount of pressure on the individual to conform to the group norms. The peer group has the greatest influence on the individual during his adolescence. For example, some of the informal aspects of culture like fashions, food, craze, etc. and forbidden knowledge, like knowledge of sex relations are acquired from the peer group.
4. *Church or Religion*—The history of man shows that religion is one of the most intimate urges of man, which is found everywhere. It is a dynamic belief and a submissive attitude to God or Gods, as supernatural beings, on whom man feels dependent. It is therefore, one of the most influential forces of society, controlling man's behaviors and socializing him. In modern societies, the importance of religion may be less. But still, it has a great influence in moulding the beliefs and ways of life. Most families observe some kind of religious practices, which are passed on to the next generation as a way of their life. A child growing up in such an environment is going to be greatly influenced by it. It will be responsible in shaping the ideas and life. Thus, it becomes an important agency of socialization.
5. *The State*—The state is a special organization of society to attain establishment of law and order. It is an instrument of the society to maintain law and order so that man can have a good life. Man has to obey the laws of the state and if he fails to obey them, he can be punished because they have the sanction of force behind them. Thus, it is an authoritarian agency of socialization, which moulds the behaviour of man.

## Types of Socialization

Ian Robertson has classified socialization into four types in his book "Sociology". According to him, the socialization that a person undergoes during his lifetime may be of one or more of the following types:
1. *Primary Socialization*—The most essential and basic type of socialization is called primary socialization. It takes place in the early years of the life of the new born individual through primary

agencies like family, friends and playmates. Primary socialization concentrates on teaching of language, cognitive skills, cultural norms, values, emotional ties and appreciation of roles and perspectives.

"Internalization of norms" is the most important aspect of primary socialization. It is a process through which norms of society become a part of the personality of the individual. The human child does not have a sense of right or wrong, desirable or undesirable, moral or immoral, at birth. The child gradually learns the norms by trial and error, by direct and indirect observation and experience. The different agencies of socialization reinforce the child's learning by rewards and punishments or by means of approval and disapproval.

2. *Anticipatory Socialization*—Individuals learn not only the culture of their own group but also learn the culture of other groups to which they do not belong. Sociologists like Merton called this as anticipatory socialization. It is a process, where by, men socialize themselves into the culture of a group with the anticipation of joining that group, for example, a person who intends to join the army may start doing physical exercises to toughen his body. He also starts learning the manners of army personnel to become one with them later on. People may be socialized into groups of which they are already members or into groups to which they wish to become attached. Thus, socialization is not a process that takes place only in early childhood, but it goes on at different times and different places throughout the life of the individual.

3. *Developmental Socialization*—Developmental socialization is based on the already acquired socialization through the primary agencies of socialization. It builds on the acquired knowledge and skills as the adult progresses through new situations, such as marriage or new jobs. It requires new expectations, obligations and roles. New knowledge will be added to make the individuals to adapt to the new situations. This new learning is added and blended with the old one in a relatively smooth and continuous process of development.

4. *Resocialization*—Individuals keep changing their roles within the groups. They also change their memberships in groups sometimes. In some cases the earlier learned patterns have to be given up and

new ones must be substituted for them to adjust to the changing roles. This is called resocialization. Such resocialization takes place when a social role is radically changed. It may also happen in periods of rapid social mobility. For example, a newly wedded woman may be forced to become a prostitute in a brothel. In this case, the social role of the woman changes radically.

## Individualization

According to Mac Iver, individualization is the process in which men become more autonomous or self-determining. It is a process by which an individual becomes independent of his group. It is a process in which man comes to know himself and acquire a sense of inner responsibility. He starts doing things because his self-approves of it. Individuality becomes his quality. Socialization brings man into relation with others whereas individualization makes him autonomous or more independent of his group or self-determining. It creates a self-consciousness in man. Socialization is a process of attaining to one's own self, when a man does things not simply because others do the same things but because his own self-approves it. He is carried by his own individuality. Thus, the following are the aspects of individualization:

1. Process of becoming different from other people.
2. Isolated people develop a different type of personality.
3. Democratization, free competition and social mobility also further individualization.
4. Becoming aware of one's own specific character and the rise of a new kind of self-evaluation. It is a feeling of self- glorification.
5. Individualization of wishes through objects, social mobility and family conditions, shape the wishes of the individual.
6. Development of a feeling of privacy and partial isolation, results in introspection, which leads to individualization.

### POINTS TO NOTE
1. Definition and meaning of basic concepts of man as a social animal.
2. Society–community-association-institutions-socialization–individualization.

## Man and Society

### NURSING IMPLICATIONS

Man being a social animal belongs to number of group like society- community- associations which are responsible for the socialization of the individual. A study of these groups gives a better understanding of the patient's behavior.

### QUESTIONS

1. Explain the process of socialization.
2. Agencies of socialization.
3. Individualization.
4. Define socialization.
5. Relation between individual and socialization.
6. What is socialization? What are stages in socialization of an individual?
7. Explain the types of socialization.
8. What is social interaction?
9. "Man is a social animal", Comment.
10. Define society. Briefly explain its characteristics.
11. What is a community? Explain its characteristics.
12. Explain the characteristics of associations.
13. Define institutions. What are its characteristics?
14. Differentiate or distinguish between:
    A. Community and association.
    B. Community and society.
    C. Association and institution.
    D. Community and institution.

new ones must be substituted for them to adjust to the changing roles. This is called resocialization. Such resocialization takes place when a social role is radically changed. It may also happen in periods of rapid social mobility. For example, a newly wedded woman may be forced to become a prostitute in a brothel. In this case, the social role of the woman changes radically.

## Individualization

According to Mac Iver, individualization is the process in which men become more autonomous or self-determining. It is a process by which an individual becomes independent of his group. It is a process in which man comes to know himself and acquire a sense of inner responsibility. He starts doing things because his self-approves of it. Individuality becomes his quality. Socialization brings man into relation with others whereas individualization makes him autonomous or more independent of his group or self-determining. It creates a self-consciousness in man. Socialization is a process of attaining to one's own self, when a man does things not simply because others do the same things but because his own self-approves it. He is carried by his own individuality. Thus, the following are the aspects of individualization:

1. Process of becoming different from other people.
2. Isolated people develop a different type of personality.
3. Democratization, free competition and social mobility also further individualization.
4. Becoming aware of one's own specific character and the rise of a new kind of self-evaluation. It is a feeling of self- glorification.
5. Individualization of wishes through objects, social mobility and family conditions, shape the wishes of the individual.
6. Development of a feeling of privacy and partial isolation, results in introspection, which leads to individualization.

> **POINTS TO NOTE**
> 1. Definition and meaning of basic concepts of man as a social animal.
> 2. Society–community-association-institutions-socialization–individualization.

## Man and Society

### NURSING IMPLICATIONS

Man being a social animal belongs to number of group like society- community- associations which are responsible for the socialization of the individual. A study of these groups gives a better understanding of the patient's behavior.

### QUESTIONS

1. Explain the process of socialization.
2. Agencies of socialization.
3. Individualization.
4. Define socialization.
5. Relation between individual and socialization.
6. What is socialization? What are stages in socialization of an individual?
7. Explain the types of socialization.
8. What is social interaction?
9. "Man is a social animal", Comment.
10. Define society. Briefly explain its characteristics.
11. What is a community? Explain its characteristics.
12. Explain the characteristics of associations.
13. Define institutions. What are its characteristics?
14. Differentiate or distinguish between:
    A. Community and association.
    B. Community and society.
    C. Association and institution.
    D. Community and institution.

# CHAPTER 3

# Culture

- Nature of culture
- Evolution of culture
- Diversity and uniformity of culture
- Culture and socialization
- Transcultural society
- Influence on health and disease
- Influence of culture on health

The concepts of "culture" and "society" are fundamental concepts of Sociology. It is commonly used in social sciences like Psychology, Political Science and Economics. Culture is a very important concept in Anthropology. The study of any society makes it necessary to understand its culture. Society and culture therefore go together.

Culture is unique to man, which makes him different from the other lower animals. Man is not only a social being but also a cultural and rational being. The term "culture" as used in Sociology, has a different meaning from that used in common language.

Generally, an uneducated man is called as uncultured whereas an educated man is called cultured in common language. But, in Sociology culture is all that man learns as a member of the society i.e. all his acquired or learned behavior patterns. Thus, culture is unique to man. Since he alone has the capacity to learn.

## ■ DEFINITION

1. According to EB Tylor, an English Anthropologist, who coined the word "culture", it is "that complex whole, which includes knowledge, belief, art, morals, laws, customs and other capabilities and habits acquired by man as a member of the society."
2. Malinowski has defined culture as "the handiwork of man and the medium through which he achieved his ends."
3. Graham Wallas defined culture as "an accumulation of thoughts, values and objects"; it is the social heritage acquired by us from

preceding generations through learning, as distinguished from the biological heritage, which is passed on to us automatically through the genes."
4. According to R Bierstedt "culture is the complex whole that consists of everything we think and do and have as members of society."
5. HT Majumdar defines culture as "the sum total of human achievements, material, as well as nonmaterial, capable of transmission."

## ■ NATURE OR CHARACTERISTICS OF CULTURE

From the above definitions the following are the characteristics of culture:
1. *Culture is acquired or learned behavior pattern*—Any behavior pattern that is socially acquired is called as learned behavior pattern like dress habits, food habits, ways of greeting or worshipping god, etc.
2. *Culture is social and shared*—Culture is social and not an individual heritage. It is social because it develops through social interactions i.e. man becomes cultural only in the company of other human beings. Therefore, culture is shared among the members of a group. For example, the customs, traditions, values, beliefs, ideas and ideals, etc. are all shared by the members of a group. As Robert Biersted pointed out, it depends upon the group life for its existence.
3. *Culture is transmissive*—It is transmitted from one generation to the next and from one group to another. Man possesses language. It is through the means of language that he passes on what he has learnt to the next generation. It also helps him to learn and know things of the past. Culture is the total heritage.
4. *Culture is continuous and cumulative*—Culture is the social heritage of man. It is a "growing whole" which includes in itself, the achievements of the past and the present and makes provision for the future achievements of man.
5. *Culture is an integrated system*—The various aspects of culture are interconnected. For example, the value system of a society is closely connected with its other aspects, such as values, morals, religion, customs, traditions, etc.

6. *Culture is dynamic, as well as adaptive*—Culture is not static. It keeps adjusting to the changing conditions around in the society, though very slowly.
7. *Culture is gratifying*—Culture helps man to satisfy his basic needs and desires. These needs may be biological like food, shelter and clothing or social like name and fame, money, mates, etc. are all fulfilled by man according to his culture.
8. *Culture varies from society to society*—Culture varies from society to society, from group to group and from time to time. It evolves into more complex forms through the ages like the ways of eating, dressing, speaking a language, greeting, etc.
9. *Culture is idealistic*—Every culture has its own set of ideas and norms, according to which the individuals have their behavior patterns.
10. *Culture is super organic*—It is independent of physical and physiological properties and characteristics. For example, the "flag" represents a nation or professors, engineers or doctors being viewed differently in every society according to the social status and role as understood in their culture.

## ■ EVOLUTION OR DEVELOPMENT OF CULTURE

Culture is as old as mankind because man alone has culture. It is his culture, which makes him different from the other animals in the society. Culture evolved gradually over a period of time. It cannot be pointed out exactly as to when culture began but it can be said that it must have begun with man's capacity to use and to create or produce tools and techniques. The first kinds of tools used by man were in the form of stones, some five million years ago. They were used by him as weapons. He gradually learnt to use fire and some forms of language. Thus, as the biological evolution of man took place, culture also developed. The growth and development of culture can take place because of man's capacity to learn. Man alone has language and therefore, he can inhabit the past, present and future. He can accumulate culture and transmit it to the next generation. Thus, man is born in a stream of culture and must cotinuously swim in it, if he has to live as a member of the society.

## Types of Culture

Culture has been broadly distinguished as material and nonmaterial culture. These cultural factors have an influence on social change. Ogburn was the first Sociologist to use the concept of "cultural-lag" to explain social change. He made a distinction between material and nonmaterial culture. According to him, material culture is those aspects of culture which are manmade like tools, implements, machinery, houses and other utilitarian objects. These are devices and instruments by which nature is controlled and makes life more comfortable. In the nonmaterial aspects of culture, he includes religion, values, beliefs, ideas, ideals, attitudes, etc. According to him, changes in the aspect of material culture stimulate changes in the aspects of nonmaterial culture but changes in the aspects of nonmaterial culture are slow compared to the aspects of change in material culture. Therefore, nonmaterial culture falls behind the material culture and the result is a "lag" between the two. This he called as the "cultural lag". For example, in the modern industrial societies, discoveries and inventions are rapidly made, to which the nonmaterial culture has to adjust itself and if it cannot, a lag occurs. This is due to the rigidity of the ideological system. The lags that have appeared during the last few years have generally been between a rapidly advancing technology and old elements of belief and organization. In other words, man in order to remove the gaps between the two parts of culture, should adapt his ways of thinking and behaving to the state of his technology.

## ■ DIVERSITY AND UNIFORMITY OF CULTURE

As pointed out earlier, cultures differ from people to people, groups to groups and society to society. These variations have an effect on the behavior of the people. Some of the factors responsible for cultural variability are historical accidents, geographical environment, mobility of human beings, inventions and discoveries, individual peculiarities, changes in the modes of production, dominant cultural themes, etc. The above factors explain why different societies have different ways of satisfying their needs due to different environmental conditions.

Inspite of the variability in cultures, it can be said that there are cultural universals like quarrel, love, associate and procreate. The existence of such universals indicates their utility and suggests that there are practices to which a man is well adapted and has a need.

## Culture and Socialization

As observed earlier socialization is a learning process. It is a continues process which changes man from a biological being to a social and cultural being. It is through this process that man learns the culture of the society into which he is born and lives. Therefore man is dependent on socialization for learning the culture and becoming a normal human being. Culture and socialization are inter related. Culture is a social heritage of a group of people. It consists shared behavior, beliefs and material objects belonging to society. It is habits attitudes and values which are transmitted from generations to generation. Socialization is the process by which young members learn the culture if the society. This has an impact on the formation the personality of the individual.

## Transcultural Society

Transcultural is described as "extending through all human cultures" or "involving, encompassing or combing elements of more than one culture", i.e. bringing together elements of different cultures, e.g., a mothers love for her child is transcultural since it exist in all human cultures. Something that is true across all cultures can be described as transcultural. Sociologists, Anthropologies and Historians are particularly interested in things that are transcultural since they study the way humans interact in various societies cultures and time periods.

## Elements of Culture

According to HM Johnson, the main elements of culture are the following:
1. Cognitive elements consist of the knowledge about the physical and social world.
2. Beliefs in empirical terms are neither true nor false.

3. Values are measures of goodness or desirability.
4. Norms are closely related to values. They are the group shared standards of behavior.
5. Signs include signals and symbols. A signal indicates the existence - past, present or future - of a thing, event or conditions. A symbol signifies a form of something, the meaning of which is cultural.
6. Non-normative ways of behaving are certain behavior patterns, which exist and which are not normative and often unconscious. They gradually become normative and symbolic in course of time.

## ■ FUNCTIONS OF CULTURE

Man is a cultural being. He is also called as a culture creating animal. It is his culture, which differentiates him from the other animals. Culture plays an important role in the life of the individual, as well as the society. It is man's culture, which sets up certain standards of behavior for him and for the society. The following are the functions of culture:

### For the Individual

a. Culture makes man a human being. Man, born as a biological being, becomes a social being through his culture. He learns the various ways of living and satisfying his basic needs through culture i.e. the qualities required to live a social life are acquired by man through his culture.
b. Culture provides solutions for complicated situations. Culture not only helps man to conduct his life and living smoothly but it also provides him with solutions for day-to-day complicated situations. This saves him the time to think and act. Culture provides him with a set of standard behavior patterns for most situations in his daily life, like the way he has to dress, the kind of food he has to eat, etc.
c. Culture provides traditional interpretations to certain situations. Man learns to behave in certain situations according to certain traditional interpretations given by his culture. These may differ from culture to culture for example, when a cat crosses the path of an individual when he is setting out on a journey, he postpones his journey. Among some cultures, an owl is regarded as a symbol of wisdom and among some others as a symbol of idiocy.

## For the Group

a. Culture keeps social relations intact. It helps to maintain group life. Man lives in groups and his relationships in the groups are regulated by culture. Culture is the design and the prescription, the composite of guiding values. People have a standard behavior in the society because of their culture. Thus, culture has an importance not only for man but also for the society. The group solidarity rests on the group culture.
b. Culture broadens the vision of the individual. Culture brings about a change in the outlook of the individuals by providing them with a set of rules for their behavior in the society. It makes him think not only of himself but also about the others. He thinks of himself as a part of the larger society.
c. Culture creates new needs. Man has a number of needs and drives, which he satisfies through his culture. Culture creates new drives and needs. It satisfies the aesthetic, moral and religious interests of the members of the group. In this way, groups owe much to culture.

## CULTURAL FACTORS IN HEALTH AND DISEASE

Culture plays an important role in the life of the individual and the group in which he lives. It includes his beliefs, values, ideas, attitudes, ideals, traditions, customs, religious practices, etc. which influence his behavior pattern in his health and disease conditions.

These effect his food habits, nutrition and the implementation of health programs, the meaning and response to sickness and the choice of treatment. For example, a sickness may have different meanings for different people because of their tradition and culturally sanctioned beliefs and attitudes. Some diseases like leprosy or paralysis are regarded as punishment given by God in some cultures. Therefore, such people give more importance to poojas, religious ceremonies and rituals in order to satisfy the god and get out of the curse of God. Medical treatment in such cases becomes secondary to them.

The response and choice of treatment for a disease varies from person to person because of various factors in his culture. For example, in India people choose to go for herbal medicines for the treatment of jaundice. Sometimes they go in for other alternate medicine like homeopathy, naturopathy, traditional healers or home remedies.

Some cultural beliefs related to health and diseases, which are practiced in India are the following:

1. Certain diseases like chicken-pox, measles, mumps, etc., are considered to be due to the wrath of some God and Goddesses. Therefore, drugs are not given but poojas are performed to appease the Gods.
2. Drinking tulsi water or water stored in a copper vessel is good for health.
3. Purdah system followed by the Muslim women causes vitamin-D deficiency.
4. Giving an iron object during convulsions will reduce the intensity of the fits.
5. Family Planning is not practiced among some members of some communities because they believe that children are a gift of God.
6. Male child is preferred by the Hindus because of their belief that only a male child has the right to perform the last rites for his parents, who will then achieve Moksha.

Some cultural beliefs, related to food habits, practiced in India are the following:

1. Some higher caste sections among the Hindus do not consume certain food like onion, garlic, drum-sticks, and nonvegetarian foods.
2. Consuming certain food items like egg, fish, brinjal, mango, produces allergy.
3. Avoiding fatty foods in postoperative period.
4. Periodic fasting helps in the cleansing of the digestive system.
5. Beet-root consumption enhances blood production in the body.

### POINTS TO NOTE
1. Culture–nature or characteristics–types–diversity and uniformity–elements–functions.
2. Cultural factors in health and diseases.
3. Culture and socialization.
4. Trans-cultural society.

# Culture

## NURSING IMPLICATIONS

Culture being a way of life of the people, studying it becomes important for understanding behavior of patients for health care professionals especially in case of health and disease conditions. This knowledge helps them in understanding and treating of patients.

## QUESTIONS

1. Define:
    a. Culture
    b. Cultural-lag
    c. Culture and socialization
    d. Trans-cultural society
2. Give the characteristics of culture.
3. Discuss the theory of cultural-lag given by Ogburn.
4. What are the functions of culture?
5. Mention some food beliefs and their effects on health.
6. Mention some beliefs in Indian culture, which have beneficial health effects.
7. Mention some beliefs in Indian culture which have adverse health effects.
8. How does culture influence an individual?
9. What is the impact of culture on human behavior?
10. Bring out the importance of knowing the culture of a patient for the nurse.
11. Bring out the relationship between culture, health and illness.

# CHAPTER 4

# Social Processes

- Social interaction meaning definition
- Social process meaning and definition
- Cooperation
- Competition
- Conflict
- Accommodation
- Assimilation
- Isolation
- Forms of social processes-conjunctive or associative social processes
- Associative social processes-disjunctive or dissociative social processes

Society is a system of social relationships. These relationships represent the functional aspects of society. Social processes deal with the functional aspects of human association. These social processes therefore may be described as the fundamental ways in which men interact and establish relationships. They are certain repetitive forms of behavior, which are commonly found in social life. There are different types of social relationships giving rise to different types of social processes. Thus, social process is mainly dependent upon the kind of social interaction that individuals or group members have with each other. Social interaction and social processes are interrelated.

Mac Iver defined society as a "web of social relationships". Social relationships are important for man because man is sociocultural by nature. He is a gregarious being. i.e. he has the tendency to live in groups and cannot live alone. As members of the groups, they establish relationships with the others in the groups, giving rise to behavior patterns. The behavioral pattern of one individual effects the behavior of the other. Thus, behavior systems grow out of interactions. Without these interactions there cannot be any social or group life. Only people coming together do not make up a group. It is only when there is awareness and response between the individuals that a social relationship is established. Thus, interaction is the basic ingredient of social relationships. Society is rooted in social interaction. Therefore, according to Park and Burgess, the two important elements in social interaction are - social contact and communication.

## ■ DEFINITION

1. According to Elridge and Merrill "Social interaction is the general process whereby two or more persons are in meaningful contact as a result of which their behavior is modified, however slightly.
2. Green defines social interaction as "the mutual influences that individuals and groups have on one another in their attempts to solve the problems and their striving towards goals.
3. According to Gist "social interaction is the reciprocal influences human beings exert on each other through inter stimulation and response".
4. Dawson and Gettys define social interaction "as a process whereby men interpenetrate the minds of each other."

From the above definitions, social interaction means the social relationships where in there is a reciprocal stimulation and response between individuals to satisfy their needs and interests and to solve their problems. The whole society is based on social interaction. It is on the basis of social interactions that culture arises and continues to be there in the society. It is through social interaction that the process of socialization of individuals takes place. Thus, social interaction becomes a necessary condition for the existence of the society.

1. According to Horton and Hunt—Social process is "the repetitive forms of behaviors, which are commonly found in social life".
2. Mac Iver describes social process as "the manner in which the relations of members of a group, once brought together, acquire a distinctive character."
3. According to Ginsberg social processes mean "the various modes of interaction between individuals or groups, including cooperation and conflict, social differentiation and integration, development, arrest and decay."

4. According to Green A.W social process is "the characteristic ways in which interaction occurs."

All the above definitions show that the basis for social process is social interaction. There are different kinds of social processes depending upon the social relationships. Some of the important forms of social processes are cooperation, competition, conflict, accommodation, assimilation and isolation.

## FORMS OF SOCIAL PROCESSES

Social Processes can be classified as:
1. Conjunctive or associative social processes like cooperation, organization adjustment, accommodation, integration and assimilation.
2. Disjunctive or dissociative, social processes like conflict, isolation, competition, differentiation, disintegration, and contravention and war.

## ASSOCIATIVE OR CONJUNCTIVE SOCIAL PROCESSES

### Cooperation

*Meaning*

Cooperation is an associative social process. It is derived from the Latin words "co" meaning "together" and "operari" meaning "to work". Therefore, it generally means two or more persons working together for the pursuit of a common goal or objective or reward. It is the most basic and common social process for group life and for the society. It may be a small group like the family, where members have to cooperate with each other to complete the functions of the family or a larger group like a school, where again cooperation is required for the organization to function properly. The basic needs of the individual like food, shelter and clothing can be provided and satisfied only through cooperation. It is a physical, biological, psychological and social necessity of man during his life time. Thus, it is a universal and continuous social phenomenon. It is essential for economic life also. Division of labour and specialization are examples of economic cooperation.

## Definition

1. *Merrill and Elridge*—"Cooperation is a form of social interaction wherein two or more persons work together to gain a common end".
2. *Fair child*—"Cooperation is the process by which the individuals or groups combine their efforts, in a more or less organized way for the attainment of a common objective".
3. *AW Green*—"Cooperation is the continuous and common endeavor of two or more persons to perform a task or to reach a goal that is commonly cherished".

## TYPES OF COOPERATION

### Direct Cooperation

Individuals work together to achieve a common objective i.e., the members of the group have an identical function. Members do the work "in company" with others. Doing the work together gives them social satisfaction. There is a direct face-to-face contact among the members like tilling the field together or playing together or taking out a cart from the mud.

### Indirect Cooperation

Indirect cooperation is based on the principle of division of labor and specialization of skills. People do unlike jobs to achieve a common end. Each individual has his own specialized function to perform. For example, in the construction of a building, the masons, plumbers, carpenters and others, cooperate together with each other doing their specialized jobs.

### Primary Cooperation

Primary cooperation is found in primary groups like the family, peer group, neighborhood and so on. There is an identity of ends and interests between the individuals and the group. Means and goals become one for everyone. All of them work together to achieve a common end. They share the rewards of this combined effort.

### Secondary Cooperation

Secondary cooperation is found in secondary groups like industry, government, educational groups, commercial groups, religious groups, etc. In this kind of cooperation, each individual performs a specialized function. The individual members work together to achieve a common goal, but each member does a specialized task and is interested in his own gain. For example, an individual working in an industry for the gain of wages or promotions, power and prestige.

### Tertiary Cooperation

This kind of cooperation may be found between big and small groups to meet a particular situation. One is forced to cooperate with the other group due to circumstances. The attitudes of the cooperating parties are opportunistic and the organization of their cooperation is fragile and loose. This kind of cooperation may be found between two or more political parties or religious groups or caste groups and so on.

## ■ ROLE OF COOPERATION IN SOCIAL LIFE OR IMPORTANCE OF COOPERATION

Cooperation means working together for the pursuit of a common goal or objective or reward. It is one of the most basic and common form of associative social process for group life and for the society. It is a universal and continuous social phenomenon. The basic needs of the individual like food, shelter and clothing can be provided and satisfied only through cooperation. It therefore, plays a very important role in the life of the individual. His very survival in society depends on cooperation. It is a physical, biological, psychological, social and economic necessity of man during his life time. Man and Society can progress and develop only because of Cooperation. Thus, according to Prince Kropotkin it is difficult for man to survive without it. Society and man advance through cooperation and decline in its absence.

## ■ ACCOMMODATION

### Meaning

Accommodation is one of the important types of associative social processes. It is through this process that the social order and peace

Social Processes 53

is maintained. Change is the law of nature. Changes keep occurring in society and the environment around man. This may lead to a number of conflicting situations for man. There are continuous conflicts between individuals and groups. They have to therefore adjust themselves to the conflicting situations because man does not like to live in a conflicting situation. He would like to resolve them and live in peace and order. This process of adjustment of man to the social and environmental conditions around him is called accommodation. Thus, accommodation is the process of getting along with the situations that arise around man, which helps people to work together, whether they like it or not. The famous psychologist, J.M. Baldwin, first used this term to mean the changes in the behavior of individuals, which help them to adjust to their environment.

## Definition

1. *Mac Iver*—The term accommodation refers to the process in which man attains a sense of harmony with his environment.
2. *Ogburn and Nimkoff*—Accommodation is a term used by sociologists to describe the adjustment of hostile individuals or groups.
3. *Horton and Hurt*—Accommodation is a process of developing temporary working agreements between conflicting individuals or groups.
4. *Park and Burgess*—Accommodation is a natural resolution of conflicts. In accommodation, the antagonism of hostile element is for the time being regulated and conflict disappears as overt action although it remains latent as a potential.
5. *Gillin and Gillin*—Accommodation is the process by which competing and conflicting individuals and groups adjust their relationship to each other in order to overcome the difficulties, which arise in competition, contravention or conflict.

## Characteristics

1. Accommodation is the natural result of conflict. If there were no conflicts, there would be no need for accommodation. When individuals or groups have conflicts, they try to come together to solve them by a settlement. Such settlements, temporary or permanent may, be called accommodation.

2. **Accommodation is universal.** Accommodation has been found in all societies and at all times in social life. Conflicts are always there among individuals and groups in all societies. People cannot live in a state of conflicts. Therefore, people try to make adjustments in order to live in a peaceful state, which takes the form of accommodation. Thus, it becomes necessary.
3. **Accommodation is a continuous process,** where conflicting individuals and groups have to necessarily make adjustments among themselves. The process of accommodation is there throughout the life of the individual, when he has to accommodate or adjust himself to the various situations in his life. Whenever there are conflicts, sooner or later, accommodation follows.
4. **Accommodation may be conscious or unconscious.** Most of the time, the process of accommodation is unconscious i.e., man adjusts himself to the social environment around him. All through his life, man goes through the process of socialization, where he learns to live according to the norms of the society. He is controlled by the different norms of the society like the customs, traditions, morals, etc. Thus, he unconsciously learns to accommodate himself with his family, caste, class, peer group, neighborhood, work place, etc. i.e., the total social environment in which he lives. Accommodation may also be conscious where individuals or groups consciously try to make adjustments to conflicting situations. It is a deliberate attempt on the part of the individuals or groups to come together and start working together. They try to resolve their differences, for example, workers and management coming to an agreement on some conflicting issues and the workers calling off their strike by coming back to work.
5. **Accommodation is a mixture of both love and hate.** The effects of accommodation may vary with circumstances. For example, it may act to reduce conflict between persons or groups or it may serve to postpone a conflict or it may permit groups marked by sharp socio-psychological distance to get along together. In short, it may prove to be beneficial to both the parties involved.

## ■ FORMS OR METHODS OF ACCOMMODATION

Accommodation is the social process of adjustment of man and groups, to the social and environmental conditions around him, especially in conflicting situations. Gillian and Gillian have given the following forms of accommodation.

## Yielding to Coercion

Coercion is the use of or the threat of force to solve a conflict. In such cases, parties involved have an unequal strength. Generally, the stronger party uses force over the weaker party to come to an agreement and accept its terms. For example, the country, which wins the war, imposes its conditions over the vanquished country.

## Compromise

In a compromise, the parties involved are almost of equal power. In such cases, each party to the dispute makes some concessions and yields to some demands of the other. The "all or nothing" attitudes give way to a willingness to yield to certain points in order to gain others. For example, the settlement of disputes between labor and management in industry on aspects of wages, hours of work, etc. is a case of compromise.

## Arbitration

When two conflicting parties are not able to come to an agreement on their own, they take the help of a third party to come to a compromise. The decision of the third party is binding on both parties. This is called arbitration.

## Mediation

In this case, the third party i.e., a mediator only advises the conflicting parties. The mediator does not have any power to settle the conflict. His decisions are not binding on the parties. He only tries to find a solution to the problems of the conflicting parties. For example, labor-management conflicts.

## Conciliation

In conciliation, the third party tries to persuade the conflicting parties to develop friendship and come to an agreement. It is generally used to settle labor-management disputes.

## Toleration

Toleration is based on the policy of "live and let live", where there is no settlement of disputes but there is only the avoidance of overt conflict between the parties. They try to bear each other because they know that their differences are irreconcilable. Thus, they decide to co-exist with their differences. For example, the coexistence of a number of religions and religious practices in India.

## Conversion

Conversion involves a sudden rejection of one's beliefs, conviction and loyalties and adopting others views or policies or ideology. This occurs when there are differences of opinion among individuals or groups. Such conversions can be observed in religious beliefs and in the political fields.

## Rationalization

Rationalization involves plausible excuses or explanations for one's behavior i.e., the individual or party ties to justify its own behavior. They are not ready to accept their faults and shortcomings and blame others for their own behavior or faults. For example, a student may blame the school or teachers for his bad performance in the examination but will not accept his own fault of not putting in enough efforts in his studies.

## Super Ordination and Subordination

In any society, there are always relations of superiority and inferiority based on different factors. The individuals therefore have a certain fixed position or status in the society. They accept their relative positions as a matter of fact and accommodation is said to have reached a state of perfection. This is what happened in the traditional caste system of India. Such an accommodation results in harmony, friendship and sympathy between the superior and the inferior groups or individuals.

## Sublimation

Sublimation is substitution of non-aggressive attitudes and activities for aggressive ones. It may take place among individuals or groups for example, methods suggested by Jesus Christ or Gandhiji to conquer violence and hatred by love and compassion.

## ◼ ROLE OF ACCOMMODATION

Accommodation is one of the important social processes through which the social order and peace of the society is maintained. Conflicts arise in the society, which disturbs the peace and order of the society. Therefore, efforts are made in all the societies to bring about the resolution of conflicts between antagonistic groups. Accommodation checks conflict and helps persons and groups to maintain cooperation. It helps the individual to adjust himself to the changed conditions. With such adjustments, individuals are able to carry on their daily life activities inspite of different interests and points of view. Accommodation thus, becomes necessary to maintain social life. It can be at the individual or social level. Society itself is the result of accommodation.

## ◼ ASSIMILATION

Assimilation is an associative type of social process or interaction, which is also a type of adjustment like accommodation. In this process, the persons and groups acquire the culture of other groups in which they come to live, by adopting its values and attitudes, its pattern of thinking and behaving, i.e., its way of life. It requires more fundamental changes than accommodation. Assimilation is concerned with the absorption and incorporation of one culture by another. It is a process of fusion.

### Definition

1. *Biesanz*—Assimilation is the social process where by individuals or groups come to share the same sentiments and goals.
2. *Ogburn and Nimkoff*—Assimilation is the process whereby individuals or groups once dissimilar, become similar and identified in their interests and outlook.
3. *Samuel Koenig*—Assimilation is the process whereby persons and groups acquire the culture of another group.
4. *Bogardus*—Assimilation is a process whereby attitudes of many persons are united and thus develop into a united group.

5. *Horton and Hurt*—Assimilation is the process of mutual cultural diffusion through which persons and groups come to share a common culture.

## Characteristics

1. Assimilation is not confined to a single field only. It generally means the fusion of two distinct cultural groups. Assimilation can take place in any field. It is not limited to any single field. Assimilation is a process of learning like socialization. It starts when an individual comes into contact with other cultures. Assimilation is a social and psychological process. For example, children are gradually assimilated into the adult society. There can be assimilation between the husband and wife after their marriage or in the religious field, when people get converted into some other religious sect or group.
2. Assimilation is a slow and gradual process. It takes quite sometime before individuals and groups become one with each other and accept each others ways and outlook. This kind of fusion of personalities and groups usually takes time. There has to be a continuous and direct contact among them. Thus, the social contacts established finally result in assimilation. The speed of the process of assimilation depends on nature of the contacts. If the contacts are primary, assimilation occurs naturally and rapidly and if they are secondary assimilation takes place very slowly.
3. Assimilation is an unconscious process. In the process of assimilation, the individual or group is mostly unconscious of what is happening. Unknowingly many times, the individuals and groups give up their own cultural traits and adopt the new ones, when they come into contact with other cultural groups.
4. Assimilation is a two-way process. This is because it is based on the principle of give and take. This process is called as acculturation. Acculturation is the process whereby one cultural group, which is in contact with another cultural group borrows from it certain cultural elements and incorporates it into its own culture. It effects both the groups. Generally, the culturally weaker group borrows the elements of the culture of the stronger group. In course of time, it gets merged with the stronger culture. For example, the

exchanges of cultural traits between the Aryans and the Dravidians is a case of acculturation.

## Factors Favoring or Promoting Assimilation

### Toleration

Toleration helps people to come together, to develop contacts and to participate in common social and cultural activities. Assimilation becomes easy when individuals and groups are tolerant towards the cultural differences of others.

### Close Association and Intimate Social Relationships

Intimate and close social relationships help in the process of assimilation. For example, in a primary group, like the family, assimilation takes place naturally and rapidly whereas in a secondary group, it takes place very slowly because the relationships are impersonal, indirect and superficial.

### Amalgamation

Complete assimilation takes place when there is an amalgamation of individuals or groups as in the case of intergroup marriages.

### Cultural Similarity

When there are similarities in cultures, assimilation takes place quickly and at a faster rate.

### Education

Education brings about a change in the behavior of the people. Public education plays an important role in bringing about an assimilation of culture.

### Equal Social and Economic Opportunity

When people have equal social and economic opportunities, they are able to mix freely with each other, which helps in the process of assimilation.

## Factors Retarding or Hindering Assimilation

### Isolation

Close and intimate social relationships help in the process of assimilation. Isolation is a process whereby individuals or groups do not maintain any social contact or relationships. Therefore, it is a process, which hinders assimilation.

### Physical or Racial Difference

Differences in features, color of skin and other physical features may also hinder the process of assimilation.

### Cultural Differences

Cultural differences like languages, religion, customs, beliefs, etc., may also hinder the process of assimilation. This is because there are no comments among the cultures. Each group tries to maintain its own identity socially, though they may be living together physically.

### Prejudice as a Barrier to Assimilation

Prejudice segregates individuals and groups. It keeps them apart and assimilation cannot take place. Prejudice may also lead to disunity among people and groups.

### Dominance and Subordination

Domination and subordination lead to feelings of superiority and inferiority among individuals and groups. This hinders the process of assimilation.

## Distinction between Accommodation and Assimilation

1. Accommodation is not permanent whereas assimilation is permanent. There is a greater amount of adjustment among the groups in assimilation because they start identifying with each other. But in accommodation group differences are not solved permanently.
2. Accommodation may take place suddenly and in a radical manner. While assimilation is a slow and gradual process.

3. Accommodation is deliberate whereas assimilation is unconscious. Accommodation is a deliberate effort on the part of the individuals or groups to reach a settlement and therefore, it is a conscious process. But in assimilation, the individuals or groups is unconscious of what is happening. They get incorporated into another culture without becoming aware of it.

## Dissociative Social Processes

Dissociative social processes are forms of social struggle between individuals and groups. There are certain factors, which determine the positions of individuals within the groups. These processes are present in human existence and are inter-linked in a wide range of human activities. Dissociative social processes operate when the interests and attitudes are divergent. They disturb the harmonious social relationships.

## ■ COMPETITION

### Meaning

Competition is a fundamental form of dissociative social process. It is the natural result of universal struggle for existence. Cooperation and competition are always there in all societies. All people cannot satisfy all their desires. Competition is there among the human beings whenever there is an insufficient supply of things that human beings desire. It is therefore, a natural result of the universal struggle for a commodity, goal or value. For example, in the Indian society unemployment is a major social problem. Thus, there are more people seeking jobs than the jobs available. Competition can be seen in all aspects of social, economic, political and cultural life in society.

### Definition

1. *Beisanz and Beisanz*—Competition is the striving of two or more persons for the same goal, which is limited, so that all cannot share it.
2. *Horton and Hurt*—Competition is the struggle for possession of rewards, which are limited in supply like goods, status, power, love, anything.

3. *Bogardus*—Competition is a contest to obtain something, which does not exist in a quantity sufficient to meet the demand.
4. *Majumdar*—Competition is the impersonalized struggle among resembling creatures for goods and services, which are scarce or limited in quantity.

## ■ NATURE AND CHARACTERISTICS OF COMPETITION

The following characteristics of competition explain the nature of competition.
1. Competition is an impersonal struggle. It is an impersonal struggle because it is not directed against any individual or group. Most of the time, the individuals or groups competing with each other do not know each other or do not have any contact with each other. All of them only have a common aim or goal to achieve. It becomes impersonal when individuals compete with each other as members of groups as in the case of competitive examinations like the lAS or IPS or UPSC.
2. Competition is an unconscious activity. It takes place unconsciously. Many times individuals do not realize that they are competing and do not know the other competitors For example, competitive examinations, where individuals compete with each other to achieve a common goals or reward.
3. Competition is universal. It is found in all groups in all societies at all times. Competition is always there because there is always a scarcity of things that people wish to have. There is a competition at all levels - social, economic, political cultural and racial.

### Forms or Types of Competition

Bernard mentions three broad types of competitions – social, economic and political competitions.

#### *Social Competition*

A competition among people to achieve a higher status and position in the society is called social competition. Such a competition can be observed only in "open" societies, which function on democratic principles and individual merit, where talent and capacities are recognized.

## Economic Competition

Economic competition is observed in the economic processes of the society like production, distribution and consumption of goods. It can be observed among individuals and groups, when men try to achieve a higher standard of living. For example, competition for jobs, profits, wages, increments and promotions, etc.

## Political Competition

Competition is also observed in the politic field. Political parties or leaders compete with each other to secure power. This is more so during elections. There is also a keen competition among nations at international levels.

## Cultural Competition

Cultural competition may be there when there are two or more cultural groups. For example, the Aryans and the Dravidians or the Indian and the British. There may also be competition among racial groups as in the case of Negroes and Whites or between religious groups like Hindus and Muslims.

# Role or Functions of Competition

Competition is important for the society. It has a number of important and useful functions for the individual and for the society.

## Assigns Statuses to the Individuals

Competition assigns a social status to the individuals in the society. People in the society have to perform different functions, depending upon their status. Competition determines who is to perform what function, for example, division of labour in the modern complex society is a product of competition.

## Source of Motivation

Competition acts as a motivation for individuals. It makes individuals to act in a certain way to achieve certain goals or objectives. They work harder when they are competing with each other rather than on their own. It has been found that competition increases productivity.

### Conducive to Progress

Competition results in social and economic progress and the welfare of the society because it makes the individuals to work harder to achieve some goals or rewards.

### Provides for Social Mobility

Competition increases social mobility and freedom. The spirit of competition helps the individual to improve his social status.

### Provides for New Experiences

Competition provides the individuals better opportunities to satisfy their desires for new experiences and recognition.

Competition may also have its negative effects, both for the individual, as well as the society. According to Majumdar, competition may lead to neurosis through frustration; it may lead to monopoly and finally, it may lead to conflicts. Competition may create emotional disturbances. It may also create unfriendly and unfavorable attitudes among persons or groups towards one another. When competition becomes uncontrolled, it may lead to conflicts. There must therefore, always be a fair and healthy competition among people.

## Distinction between Cooperation and Competition

1. Cooperation is an associative social process where two or more persons work together to achieve a common goal or reward, while competition is a dissociative social process. It is the struggle among human beings for certain commodities, goals or values, which they desire and which are not in sufficient supply.
2. Cooperation is based on joint efforts of the people to achieve some common goals whereas competition takes place among individuals or groups to satisfy their own desire.
3. Cooperation normally results in positive results. It does not cause any loss to the individuals concerned. But competition may result in damages to the individuals or parties involved along with positive results.

4. There is no limit in cooperation because people can go to any extent to help each other, while in competition there are limitations. They have their own norms. Many times limitless or unregulated competition may result in harm or violence.
5. Cooperation requires qualities like kindness, sympathy, concern, mutual understanding and readiness to help others where as in competition qualities like strong aspirations, self-confidence, desire to earn a name and fame in society, the spirit of adventure and the readiness to suffer and to struggle are required.
6. Cooperation brings satisfaction and contentment. It lessens the internal group conflicts but competition has both positive and negative effects.

## Conflict

Conflict is a form of dissociative process. It is present in most human relations. Conflict is a form of struggle between individuals and groups. It takes place whenever a person or a group seeks to gain a reward not by surpassing other competitors but by preventing them from effectively competing.

## Definition

1. *Gillin and Gillin*—Conflict is a social process in which individuals or groups seek their ends by directly challenging the antagonist by violence or threat of violence.
2. *Horton and Hurt*—Conflict may be defined as a process of seeking to monopolize rewards by eliminating or weakening the competitors.
3. *AW Green*—Conflict is the deliberate attempt to oppose, resist or coerce the will of another or others.
4. *Majumdar*—Conflict is an opposition or struggle involving
    a. An emotional hostile attitude, as well as.
    b. A violent interference with one's autonomous choice.

Thus, conflict is a universal process. It arises primarily from a clash of interests within groups and societies and between groups and societies, as well as between individuals. It is an extreme form of competition.

## NATURE AND CHARACTERISTICS OF CONFLICT

1. *Conflict is universal*—Conflicts or clashes are present in all societies at all times. These conflicts may be very acute and vigorous in some societies and in others they may be mild.
2. *Conflict is a conscious action*—Individuals and groups that involve in conflicts are conscious of their actions. It therefore, involves deep emotions and strong passions.
3. *Conflict is personal*—When competition becomes personal, it leads to conflicts. In the struggle to overcome a group or individual, the goal becomes secondary in a conflict.
4. *Conflict is not continuous*—Conflict is not continuous. It takes place with breaks because no society can live in a state of conflict.
5. *Conflict defines issues*—Conflicts may arise between social classes, religious, social, political, economic groups and nations. The patterns of conflict changes with a change in values, attitudes, ideas, ideals, ideologies, national interests and so on.
6. *Conflict is conditioned by culture*—Conflict gets affected by the culture of the people, forcing the group. The objects of conflict may be property, power and status, freedom of action and thought or any other highly desired value.
7. *Conflicts and norms*—Norms are the social controls of the society. These norms affect the conflicts in the society.
8. *Conflict may be personal or impersonal*—Conflicts may take different forms. It may be at personal levels or at impersonal levels.
9. *Ways of resolving conflicts*—Conflicts can be resolved through the process of accommodation and assimilation.
10. *Frustration and insecurity promote conflicts*—Frustrations and insecurity lead to conflicts in the society. Individuals feel frustrated when they are not able to reach their goals.

### Forms or Types of Conflicts

Different Sociologists have classified conflicts into different types.
1. George Simmel distinguished four types of conflicts.
    i. *War*—Simmel attributed war to a deep-seated antagonistic impulse in man. The desire to gain material interest is the objective. The antagonistic impulse provides a foundation for group conflict.

ii. *Feud*—Feud is an intra-group conflict which arises due to some injustice alleged to have been done by one group to another.
iii. *Litigation*—Litigation is a judicial struggle by an individual or group to protect their right to possessions.
iv. *Conflict of impersonal ideals*—Conflict of impersonal ideals is a conflict carried on by individuals not for themselves but for an ideal. In such a conflict, each party tries to justify its own ideals, for example, the conflict carried on by the communists and capitalists is to prove that their own system can bring in a better world.

2. Gillin and Gillin have mentioned the following types of conflicts.
    i. *Personal Conflict*—Personal conflict is a conflict between two persons in the same group. For example, conflict between two students.
    ii. *Racial Conflict*—Racial conflict is conflict between two races as in the case of the whites and the Negroes in the USA.
    iii. *Class Conflict*—Class Conflict is the conflict between two classes like the employers and the employees.
    iv. *Political Conflict*—Political conflict is a conflict between political parties for political power like the conflict between the ruling party and the opposition party in the society.
    v. *International Conflict*—International conflict is a conflict between nations, for example, the conflict between India and Pakistan over the Kashmir issue.

Besides the above mentioned types of conflicts, there are also some other types of conflicts observed in the society.
    i. *Latent and Overt Conflict*—Latent conflict exists in the form of social tensions and dissatisfactions. When an issue is declared as hostile and an action is taken, the latent conflict becomes an overt conflict.
    The latent conflict between China and India may take an overt form when a war breaks out on the border issue.
    ii. *Corporate and Personal Conflict*—Corporate conflict occurs among groups within a society or between two societies, when one group tries to impose its will on the other. For example, labor management conflicts.

Personal conflict occurs within the group, though the group has very little to gain from the internal conflicts or quarrels among its members. Such conflicts may arise due to various motives, envy, hostility, betrayal of trust, etc.

## ROLE OF CONFLICT

Conflict is a fundamental human and societal trait. Conflict has both positive and negative effects.

### Positive Effects of Conflict

All conflicts need not necessarily have a bad effect. According to some sociologists like Ratzenhofer and Gumplowicz "conflict is the social process underlying social evolution and social progress. The development of societies is marked by a ceaseless struggle". Some of the positive effects of conflict are the following:

i. A limited amount of internal conflict helps to maintain the group stability. Occasional conflict among the members of a group helps in keeping the leaders of the group alert and its policies up-to-date.

ii. External conflict brings about social unity and oneness among the members of different groups to achieve a common aim. For example, during a crisis like a war, all political parties join together to help and support the government in facing the conflicts like the Indo-China War, when all the political parties came together to help the Government of India.

iii. Personal conflicts are conflicts between individuals. They are good for the individuals because they help the individual to rise to a higher level. This kind of personal opposition helps to continue the relationship.

### Negative Effects of Conflict

Conflict has negative effects also. It involves deep passions and strong emotions. Some of the negative effects of conflict are the following:

i. It disrupts social unity. It is a costly way of settling disputes. Conflicts lower the morale and weaken the solidarity of the group.

ii. It causes social disorder, chaos and confusion. History shows how wars as a form of conflict cause human and property destruction. It brings about damage and suffering for the people, which has resulted in new fears and anxieties for mankind. The fear also causes lot of psychological and moral damage. It makes the people inhuman because they would not care for human and moral values.

## Differences between Competition and Conflict

| Competition | Conflict |
|---|---|
| 1. Competition is a universal struggle for a commodity, goal or value that people desire. | Conflict is a process where a person or a group seeks to gain a reward by weakening or eliminating all rivals. |
| 2. Competition may be conscious or unconscious process. | Conflict is a conscious process. |
| 3. Competition is a universal and continuous process. | Conflict is also a universal process but not continuous. It is an intermittent process. |
| 4. Competition is impersonal because the individual is interested in achieving the goal or objective. Therefore, there is no violence involved. | Conflict is personal and may therefore take a violent form. |
| 5. Healthy competition leads to development and progress. | Conflict may lead to negative results, which is bad for the individuals, as well as society. |
| 6. Extreme form of competition leads to conflict. | Personalized competition leads to conflicts. |

## Differences between Cooperation and Conflict

| Cooperation | Conflict |
|---|---|
| 1. Cooperation is an associative social process where two or more persons work together in pursuit of a common goal or objective or reward. | Conflict is a dissociative social process where a person or a group seeks to gain a reward by weakening or eliminating all rivals. |
| 2. Cooperation may be conscious or unconscious | Conflict is a conscious deliberate act. |
| 3. In cooperation, there is sympathy, identification, kindness and a consideration for others. | In conflict, there are strong and deep emotions involved. |

*Contd...*

*Contd...*

| Cooperation | Conflict |
|---|---|
| 4. Cooperation is a universal and continuous process. | Conflict is a universal and intermittent process. |
| 5. Cooperation brings positive results. It helps in progress and development. | Conflict brings negative results, which is bad for the individual and the society. |
| 6. Cooperation is a basic social process important for society and group life. | Conflict is not necessary for group life. |

## Isolation

Man is a social animal. Social relationships are important for man because a man is a sociocultural being by nature. He is gregarious by nature and therefore has the tendency to live in groups. He cannot live alone. As members of groups, they establish relationships with each other. Without these interactions there cannot be any social or group life. According to Park and Burgess, for a social interaction there has to be a social contact and communication. The absence of social contact and communication i.e., communicative interaction is isolation. Isolation is a situation deprived of social contacts. Both the individual and the group may be isolated. It has its own effects on them.

## Types of Isolation

  i. *Absolute Isolation*—Absolute isolation is a condition where the individual has no contact with other individuals at any time.
 ii. *Spatial Isolation*—Spatial isolation is external. It is an enforced deprivation of contacts as in the case of criminals, who are imprisoned. Such individuals are deprived of any contact and protection with the outside world. Such individuals tend to become aggressive and show a greater propensity for antisocial behavior. It may lead to melancholy and other mental disorders, sexual abnormalities and antisocial attitudes.
iii. *Organic Isolation*—Organic isolation is the isolation caused by certain organic defects of the individuals, such as deafness or blindness. It is not imposed by an external force. Organic isolation is a natural condition of the individual. Such individuals

are deprived of the experiences common to healthy people. Due to their disability, they remain away from other normal human beings. They thus, lack the association by choice and the result is a narrow circle of people with whom they develop contacts. They may become suspicious, distrustful and irritable by nature. Such people may give up the hope of obtaining a normal position in life and may even become a broken personality. Organic isolation is also know as partial isolation.

iv. *Partial Isolation*—Partial isolation is an inability to make adequate responses in certain spheres of life. It may be due to some psychic reasons like a shocking childhood. It disturbs the personality of the individuals.

v. *Privacy*—Privacy also is a type of partial shyness. Privacy is a condition where the individual withdraws his inner self from the public. Excessive privacy may lead to a split-personality. It is the external circumstances, which create a set of attitudes and feelings.

vi. *Physical Isolation*—Societies may be isolated due to physical conditions like mountains, broad rivers, forests and other physical barriers, which keep them away from others in the society. Physical isolation leads to social isolation because there is a very little opportunity for the physically isolated people to come into contact with others. But with the development of means of transport and communication, the physical isolation has become less significant.

vii. *Linguistic Isolation*—Linguistic differences become barriers to social contact among people, which leads to a lack of communication among the groups. The people are unable to communicate with each other, though they may be staying together at one place.

viii. *Societal Isolation*—Sometimes isolation may be socially imposed, when a particular group prohibits its members from coming into contact with the other groups like the practice of untouchability in India. Social isolation is bad for the society as it prevents cultural borrowings. It may also be useful because it aids social solidarity on the other hand. An important consequence of this is ethnocentrism. Maintaining social distance towards other groups reinforces the integrity of particular groups. In this sense, isolation promotes the solidarity and stability of the groups.

## Social Processes

### POINTS TO NOTE

1. Definition and meaning of social processes:
   a. Cooperation
   b. Competition
   c. Conflict
   d. Accommodation
   e. Assimilation
   f. Isolation
2. Comparative study of different types of social processes and their impact on human behavior.

### NURSING IMPLICATIONS

The social processes arise out of relationships of man which have an impact on his behavior. A knowledge of these social processes helps the nurse to evaluate the patients in a better way.

### QUESTIONS

1. Define:
   a. Associative and dissociative social processes
   b. Cooperation
   c. Competition
   d. Accommodation
2. Mention the associative social processes.
3. What are the health effects of social isolation?
4. List the types of conflict.
5. What are the methods of accommodation?
6. State the functions of competition.
7. Explain the types of cooperation.
8. Write a short essay on cooperation.
9. Enumerate the social processes and their uses in society.
10. Define social processes. Explain the functional significance of cooperation, competition and conflict as social processes.
11. Write briefly about the important social processes and their significance in social system.
12. Explain the importance of cooperation in social life.
13. Distinguish between
    a. Accommodation and assimilation.
    b. Competition and conflict.
    c. Cooperation and conflict.

# CHAPTER 5

# Social Groups

- The meaning of group
- Classification of groups
- Primary and secondary groups
- In-groups verses outgroups
- Clan or sib-tribe-crowd-public and audience

Sociology is defined as the science of society and society is broadly defined as a "web of social relationships". Social relationships are the social contacts that man has with the other men around him. These social relationships give rise to groups.

Man is gregarious by nature. He has the tendency to live in groups. Society is an example of a group. It can be said to be consisting of a number of groups. A group is formed whenever two or more people get together in a meaningful way i.e., there is a social interaction or social relationship between them. Society is made up of all these social interactions. A social interaction is one where the members are aware of each other and respond to each other. These social interaction or social relationships may be of different types like friendly or unfriendly, intimate or non-intimate, inclusive or non-inclusive, specialized or non-specialized and so on. The different kinds of groups will be classified on the basis of these different relationships.

Man cannot live alone. It is only in the company of other men that man becomes social. He needs to live with other men to develop into a normal human being. The man is dependent on others to fulfill his daily needs from the time of his birth till his death. He is born into a group i.e, family and continues to be a member of a number of groups. Thus, group life becomes important for him in the society throughout his life.

## MEANING

The word "group" is used in common language also. It is used very loosely many times in Sociology also. For example, it may be used to refer to the entire society and sometimes it may be used to mean a very small group like two people coming together. Therefore, there is no specification for the group, and hence, it becomes difficult to give a single definition for the term.

### Definition

1. *Harry M Johnson*—Social group is a system of social inter-action.
2. *Mac Iver and Page*—Social group is any collection of human beings who are brought into human relationships with one another.
3. *Horton and Hunt*—Groups are aggregates or categories of people who have a consciousness of membership or interaction.
4. *Bogardus*—Social group is a collection of number of persons, two or more, who have common objects of attention, stimulating to each other, who have common loyalty and participate in similar activities.
5. *Ogburn and Nimkoff*—Social group is formed whenever two or more individuals come together and influence one another.

## CHARACTERISTICS OF SOCIAL GROUPS

From the above definitions, it can be said that the following are the important characteristics of the social groups:
1. *Collection of Individuals*—There must be at least two or more people to form a group. Without individuals there cannot be a group. The size of the group will have its impact on its members.
2. *Reciprocal Relations*—The members of the group must have a relationship with each other. They must interact or respond with each other i.e., they have a reciprocal relationship.
3. *Mutual Awareness*—The members of the group not only interact with each other but they must also be aware of each other. The behavior of the members depends upon this mutual awareness and mutual recognition of each other.
4. *Sense of Unity and Solidarity*—There is a strong sense of unity and solidarity among the members of a group because of the

frequent and constant interaction among the members. This unity is maintained consciously by the members.
5. *Common Interests*—The members of a group share common interests and goals. They work together to satisfy them.
6. *We-feeling*—The common interests and goals of the group brings the members together. This leads to emotional closeness among the members. Thus, a "we" feeling grows among them. "We" feeling is the tendency on the part of the members to identify themselves with the groups.
7. *Similar Behavior*—The members of a group have a similar behavior because they have a common interest and goal.
8. *Group norms*—Every group has its own rules and regulations or norms for its functioning, which the members are supposed to follow.
9. *Groups are Dynamic*—Groups are not static. They are dynamic. There are continuous changes in the group.
10. *Stability*—Groups may be stable or unstable and permanent or temporary.
11. *Influence on the Personality*—Groups have an influence on the personality of the individual because different types of groups act as socializing agents for the individual.

From the above important characteristics of social groups, it becomes clear that social groups are very important for the very existence and survival of the man in the society. Man is born as a biological being. He becomes a social and a cultural being only in the company of other human beings. This is also evident from the various studies of human beings that did not develop human characteristics in the absence of human beings around him, like the case of the two wolf children found in a wolf den - one was eight and the other about two years old. The younger child died immediately after it was discovered. The elder one, named Kamala had not developed any of the human traits of a normal child of her age would. She had learnt to walk on her "fours" i.e., two hands and two legs. She had not learnt any language. It was only at a later stage, when she was in the company of other human beings that she learnt some of the normal human behavior patterns. There was also another such case of isolation of an American child Anna, an illegitimate child, from the age of six months. After five years, when she was found, it was observed that she had not developed any of the normal traits of a child of that age, like walking or talking.

These cases show that man is dependent on the groups for the development of his personality. He cannot develop in isolation. Man's physical, social, emotional and psychological development takes place only through the groups.

## ■ CLASSIFICATION OF SOCIAL GROUPS

Sociologists have classified social groups into different types on different basis. They have classified them on the basis of size, nature of relations of the members forming the groups, degree of organization, kind of interests of the group and so on. Some of the classifications of social groups are the following:

1. *Charles Cooley*—Primary and secondary-relationships
2. *WG Sumner*—In - groups and out - groups - group feelings
3. *G Simmel*—Single person-nomad, dyad, triad and so on - size
4. *Tonnies*—Gemeinschaft and Gessellschaft
5. *FH Giddings*—Genetic and congregate

| Sociologist | Groups | Basis of classification |
| --- | --- | --- |
| CH Cooley | 1. Primary—Family<br>2. Secondary—School | Relationships of the individuals |
| WG Sumner | 1. In-groups-family<br>2. Out-group—"they" feeling | Individual's identification with group or feeling of belonging to a group. |
| George Simmel | 1. Small groups—like a dyad, triads and so on.<br>2. Large groups—like political party, nation. | Size |
| Dwight Sanderson | 1. Voluntary—like joining a club on his own.<br>2. Involuntary—like being a member of the family.<br>3. Delegate—joins as a representative of a number of people. | Structure |

*Contd...*

*Contd...*

| Sociologist | Groups | Basis of classification |
|---|---|---|
| Ferdinand Tonnies | 1. Gemeinschaft i.e., a community like family or village, where relationships are very intimate and close.<br>2. Gessellschaft i.e., an association where people come together to satisfy their needs and interests. No intimate relationships. | Relationship |
| FH Griddings | 1. Genetic—like the family into which man is born and becomes a member involuntarily.<br>2. Congregate—a voluntary group that man joins on his own like an office. | Membership |
| PA Sorokin | 1. Horizontal groups—large groups like the nation and political party.<br>2. Vertical groups—smaller groups like caste or class in the society. | Size |
| Charles Ellwood | 1. Involuntary groups like family.<br>2. Voluntary groups like the trade union.<br>3. Institutional groups like the church, which are mostly permanent in nature.<br>4. Non-institutional groups like the crowd which are temporary in nature. | Nature |
| Park and Burgess | 1. Territorial groups like the state or community.<br>2. Non-territorial groups like caste or class. | Geographical area |

*Contd...*

Contd...

| Sociologist | Groups | Basis of classification |
|---|---|---|
| Leopold Von Wiese and Howard Becker | 1. Crowds is an example of a temporary group, which forms suddenly. It is also an example of an unorganized group.<br>2. Groups are collection of individuals, which are more permanent.<br>3. Collectivities—abstract collection like a state or a church. | Structure and nature |

Groups are also classified as organized and unorganized groups, formal and informal groups, majority and minority groups, independent and dependent groups, open and closed groups, congregated and dispersed groups and so on.

# CH COOLEY'S CLASSIFICATION OF SOCIAL GROUPS

## Primary and Secondary Groups

CH Cooley has classified social groups as primary and secondary groups on the basis of the nature and character of the social interaction i.e., the nature of social contact and the degree of intimacy among the members of the group.

## Characteristics of the Primary Groups

Some of the important characteristics of the primary groups are the following:
1. *Size*—The primary group is small in size. The number of members making up the group is small.
2. *Physical Proximity*—The size of the primary group being small, the members are able to have a very close relationship and contact with each other. Also, there is a face-to-face contact, a physical closeness among the members of the group. This also results in intimate relations among them as in the case of the

family or peer group or neighborhood. This direct face-to-face contact also helps the members to have good communication among them.
3. *Stability*—The social relationships in the primary group are intimate and personal. Therefore, they are long lasting and the members develop a sense of "we" feeling. Thus, they are relatively more permanent and stable like the family.
4. *Intensity of Shared Interests*—The members of the primary group have and share common interests, which sustains the group. They cooperate with each other to achieve their interest.

## Importance of Primary Groups

Primary groups are very important for the individual, as well as the society.

### For the Individual

1. The primary groups play a very important role in socializing the individual. They are responsible for changing the biological being into a human being. For example, the family, the peer-group or the neighborhood play an important role in the socialization of the individual and the development of the personality of the individual.
2. *Satisfaction of Psychological Needs*—Man is not only a social being but also a psychological being. His psychological need for love, affection, sympathy are satisfied in the primary group alone, because here he has the advantages of having a close relationship with the members of the group.
3. *Provision of a Stimulus*—The persons of a primary group have common interest and therefore work together to achieve them. Thus, it acts as a stimulus for the members. Each individual gets help, inspiration and cooperation from others. There is unity among the members. All of them work together to achieve their interests.

### For the Society

1. The spirit and desire for democracy and freedom is developed in the primary groups, which is essential for the society.

2. The primary groups like the family, the peer group, neighborhood, etc. act as agents of social control. They are thus helpful for the society as they control the behavior of the individuals in the society.

## Secondary Groups

The secondary groups are exactly the opposite of the primary groups. The primary groups are enough to satisfy the needs of people in simple societies. But as the societies become more modern, complex and industrial, the secondary groups become a necessity in the society because they satisfy some important needs and interests of the individual, as well as the society. Mac Iver and Page therefore refer to them as "the great associations" For example, the factory, the labor union, the state, the church, etc.

## Characteristics of the Secondary Groups

Some of the important characteristics of the secondary groups are the following:

1. *Size*—The secondary groups are large in size. The number of members making up the group is large and may be spread over a large area like political parties or the Lions Club or Rotary Club, etc.
2. *Membership*—Membership in the secondary groups are voluntary and not compulsory. An individual is free to join any secondary group like a political group or an association or a club, according to his needs and interests.
3. *No Physical Closeness*—The secondary groups are large in size, with no definite area. There is no physical closeness among its members as in the case of the Lions Club or the Rotary Club. Therefore, there is indirect communication among the members. The social relations are impersonal, indirect and formal. The relations exist among the members till such time they satisfy their needs and interests.
4. *Social Control*—Formal means of social control like laws, police, courts, etc. are required to control the behavior of the members because the size of the group is very large and spread over a wide area.

5. *Group Structure*—The secondary groups are formed for a certain purpose like a school or a hospital. Therefore, they have a formal structure, where each individual has a specified status and role in the organization. Secondary groups are an example of organized groups. They are also called as "special interest groups".
6. *Limited Influence on Individual*—An individual's involvement in the secondary groups is limited because he spends much less time in the secondary groups. Thus, they have a limited influence on the personality of the individual.

## Importance of Secondary Groups

The secondary groups become important for the individual and the society, as the society becomes complex, modern and industrial. The needs and interest of man become more varied, which cannot be satisfied by the primary groups. He starts depending on the secondary groups for satisfying many of his needs and interests. Man has therefore started showing a great loyalty towards the secondary groups.

Secondary groups have brought about greater efficiency in the society since they work on the principle of division of labour. This has also opened up a number of opportunities for the people, where individual talents can be developed. It also broadens the outlook of the members. Thus, the secondary groups become important for the individual, as well as the society.

## Differences between Primary and Secondary Groups

| Primary groups | Secondary groups |
| --- | --- |
| Size of the group is small and limited to a particular area. | Size of the group is large and widely spread over a large area. |
| Primary groups are groups, which have a direct, face-to-face, intimate and personal relationships. | Secondary groups have indirect, not intimate and impersonal relationships. |
| There is physical proximity and direct face-to-face communication among the members. | There is no physical proximity and direct face-to-face communication among the members. |
| Interests of the members are general. | Secondary group are formed for achieving or satisfying certain aims or interests. Thus, there are specific |

*Contd...*

*Contd...*

| Primary groups | Secondary groups |
|---|---|
|  | interests in every secondary group. Therefore, they are also called as "special interest groups." |
| Relationship is not for any purpose. | Relationship is for a definite purpose. |
| There is spontaneous cooperation among the members. | There is cooperation among the members for the achievement of their aims or objectives for which the group is formed. It is not spontaneous but deliberate cooperation. |
| Primary groups are more stable and durable. | Secondary groups may be temporary or permanent. |
| Primary groups are unorganized and therefore have an informal structure. | Secondary groups are organized for a specific purpose. They have a set of rules for their organization and therefore have a formal structure. |
| Primary groups have a great influence on the individual members personality development. | Secondary groups do not have much influence on the individual members. |
| Primary groups have a strong social control over its members. Informal means of social controls are enough to control the individual's behaviors. | Secondary groups do not have a very strong control over its members. Therefore, formal social controls are required to control the individual's behaviors. |

WG Sumner, an American Sociologist has classified groups as ingroups and outgroups on the basis of the individual's identification with a group. i.e., his feeling of belonging to a group. Therefore, an ingroup is a "we-group" and an outgroup is a "they group". For example, the group to which an individual belongs, like his family, is an example of an ingroup and other families become his outgroups.

An outgroup is therefore, defined by the individual in relation to his ingroup. The outgroup for him is the group towards which he feels a sense of indifference, avoidance, disgust competition, etc.

An individual belongs to a number of social groups in the modern complex societies. The membership in these groups is overlapping.

Therefore, there is the possibility of a number of his ingroup and outgroup relationships overlapping.

The members of an ingroup identify themselves with the other members of the group and also with the group. A feeling of belonging to the group develops among the ingroup members. In such groups there is cooperation, goodwill, mutual help and respect for one another among the members. There is a sense of solidarity, loyalty, friendliness, a feeling of cooperation, of brotherhood and readiness to sacrifice themselves for the group among the members.

These feelings of ingroup members sets them apart from the other groups in the society, which become their outgroups. The attitudes of an individual towards the outgroup members is one of antipathy, which may range from a mild dislike to one of intense hatred, which would be visible in their behavior towards the outgroup members.

## ■ ETHNOCENTRISM

Ethnocentrism is an outcome of the characteristic of ingroups. According to Sumner, ethnocentrism is "that view of things in which one's own group is the center of everything and others are scaled and rated with reference to it". Every individual and every group has this ethnocentric attitude. It is the way an individual or group looks at those people or groups belonging to another group. They tend to compare themselves or their groups with others and in the process, tend to think that their own group, their culture, their attitudes and values are the best or more superior to the others. These feelings effect the behaviors of people towards the other groups and in extreme cases may also lead to hatred and contempt for them. Though ethnocentrism brings about cooperation and solidarity among the ingroup members because of their identification with the group, it may come in the way of inter group cooperation and mutual understanding. It may thus become harmful for the individual and the society.

### Spatial Groups

The spatial groups are those which are constituted because of their spatial contiguity of their members, such as the clan or sib, tribe and band, etc.

## Clan or Sib

A clan or sib is generally a part of the tribal group. It consists of blood relations either from the father's or mother's lineage and all the offsprings of one ancestor. The ancestor is supposed to be the founder of the clan. All the descendents are known by his name. It does not consist of lineages of both the father and the mother. Its descendents are either patrilineal or matrilineal. Thus, it is unilateral and exogamous. According to Majumdar, "a clan or a sib is often the combination of a few lineages and descent, who may be ultimately traced to a mythical ancestor, who may be human, animal, plant or even inanimate." Thus, it can be said that a clan is a collection of unilateral families, whose members believe themselves to be the common descendents of a real or mythical ancestor.

## Characteristics or Features of a Clan

1. *Exogamous Group*—A clan is an exogenous group i.e., an individual does not marry an individual of his own clan since they are supposed to be the descendents of the same ancestor.
2. *Common Ancestor*—The members of a clan have a common ancestor, which may be real or mythical and through whom they trace their lineage and descent.
3. *Unilateral Group*—A clan consists of all the relatives of either the father's or mother's lineage i.e., descendents are either partitineal or matrilineal. Thus, it is unilateral.

## Functions of a Clan

The functions of the clan are:
1. *Mutual Assistance and Protection*—The members of a clan have a "we feeling" because of their common lineage and descent. Therefore, they are prepared to assist and protect each other.
2. *Control Over the Members*—The clan has a great control over its members. Thus, antisocial activities of the members are controlled and the peace and order maintained within the clan. The disputes and conflicts among the members are settled by the head of the clan. Thus, it performs an administrative, as well as a legal function.
3. *Religious Function*—The clan also caters to the religious needs of its members. Usually, the head of the clan is also its priest.

## Tribe

Tribe is a social group living in a definite common geographical area, with a common name, common dialect, common religion and a common culture. Generally, they are all blood-relations living together and having their own political organization.

According to George Peter Murdock, a tribe is a "social group in which there are many clans, nomadic bands, villages or other sub-groups, which usually have a definite geographical area, separate language, singular and distinct culture and either a common political organization or at least a feeling of common determination against strangers." The Imperial Gazette of India defines a tribe as "a group of families bearing a common name, speaking a common dialect, occupying or professing to occupy a common territory and is not usually endogamous, though originally it might have been so."

## Characteristics of a Tribe

1. *Common Territory*—The tribe generally lives in a definite geographical area.
2. *Sense of Unity*—The members of a tribe have a sense of unity since they live together in the same area.
3. *Common Language*—The members of a tribe have a common language, with a dialect of their own.
4. *Endogamous*—Tribe is an endogamous group i.e., they marry within their own group.
5. *Blood Relationship*—The members of a tribe are blood relations and they draw their descent through a common ancestor, which may be real or mythical.
6. *Political Organization*—Tribe has its own political organization, with a chief, who exercises control over all the members of the tribe. He has an important place in the tribe. He is responsible for solving the problems of the group and for the protection of its members.
7. *Importance of Religion*—Religion has a very important place in the tribal organization. Members of the tribe worship a common ancestor.
8. *Common name and Culture*—The members of a tribe consider themselves to be the descendents of a common ancestor. Therefore they have a common name and a common culture.

## Distinction between Tribe and Clan

| Tribe | Clan |
|---|---|
| Tribe lives in a definite common geographical area. | Clan has no definite territory. |
| Tribe has a common language. | Clan has no common language. |
| Tribe is an endogamous group. | Clan is an exogamous group. |

## Mob

A mob is a large or disorderly crowd bent on riotous or destructive action it is generally an angry crowd that could easily become violent. A mob generally takes the law into their hands, it is a group which gathers temporarily for a particular reason. It is also sometimes described as an organized crime. There are chances of destruction, damage to property and a threat to people lives it can influence and change peoples behavior it may also live to anti-social behavior.

## Crowd

Crowd is an unorganized, temporary social group whose members are in close proximity with each other and whose object may be of diverse kinds. There are different types of crowd, which vary from each other.

## Definition

1. Mac Iver defines a crowd as "a gathering of a considerable number of people around a center and a common point of attraction."
2. According to Horton and Hunt a crowd is "a temporary collection of people reacting together to a stimuli."

## Characteristics of a Crowd

1. *Physical Presence*—Crowd is a physical presence of people. Without the presence of the people being physically present, there cannot be a crowd.
2. *Temporary*—Crowd is a temporary social group because the people cannot be present for a very long time at a given time and place. It is a transitory situation, which comes into existence due

to a certain "occasion" and comes to an end as soon as the purpose is realized.
3. *Unorganized*—Crowd is unorganized because a certain occasion or situation may give rise to a crowd. It forms suddenly and also dies off suddenly.
4. *Anonymity*—People in a crowd have a feeling of anonymity because of its unorganized nature. The individuals do not know each other in a crowd, which may lead to irresponsible behavior of the individuals.
5. *Suggestibility*—The members of a crowd are highly emotional and excited. They are easily carried away by feelings, emotions, actions, opinions of the others in the group. Thus, people in a crowd are said to be highly suggestible.
6. *Spontaneity*—Crowd is formed spontaneously and the behavior of the members is also spontaneous, which may results in an impulsive behavior.
7. *Invulnerability*—The members of a crowd do not have the hold of social control over them since they lack self-consciousness and responsibility. They are not recognized and therefore, they behave irresponsibly.

## Public

Public is an unorganized social group. It consists of people who share some common opinion, common desire or common interest. They are scattered over a large area.

## Definition

1. According to Horton and Hurt "a public is a scattered group of people, who share an interest in a particular topic."
2. Ginsberg defines public as "an unorganized aggregation of persons, who are bound together by common opinions, desires, but are too numerous for each to maintain personal relation with others."

## Characteristics of Public

1. *Dispersed Group*—Public is a dispersed group because the members do not have a direct contact with each other. Members

interact with each other only through the mass media. Therefore, the relationships among the members are indirect, impersonal and not intimate.
2. *Definite Issue*—A definite issue brings the public into existence. All people who have an interest in the same issue come to form the public.
3. *Deliberative Group*—It is a discussion group. The interaction among the members is based on discussion, deliberation, debate, disapproval, criticism, exchange of ideas, etc.
4. *Lack of Organization*—Public does not have any organization. It is a kind of a shapeless group, whose size and membership keeps changing with the change in issues.
5. *Rational Group*—It is based on rational principles. There is scope for debate, discussion, etc. It is bound by norms and therefore, people's behavior is more controlled.

## Audience

Audience is a kind of collective behavior. It is an institutionalized passive crowd. Kimbal Young defines it as "a crowd formed for a specific period of time based on some specific laws."

## Characteristics of Audience

1. People come together at a particular place to share some common purpose or interest, e.g., people coming together in a theater to see a drama or movie.
2. There is a predetermined time and place for the audience i.e. people getting together to listen to a lecture in a lecture-hall.
3. There is a standard code of behavior for the audience. For example, clapping at an appropriate time only.
4. There is a standard form of polarization and interaction between the performer and the audience. Polarization is the "mental unity of the crowd." For e.g., the audience in a magic show is a polarized crowd because each person is facing the magician on the stage. On this basis, the audience may be differentiated as a "causal" audience and a "scheduled" audience. A "causal" audience is that group of people that come together accidentally and become polarized e.g., a street play. A "scheduled" audience is that group of people who assemble at a particular place and at a fixed time.

It is more conventionalized and less spontaneous. For example, people coming together to listen to the lecture of a political leader at a maidan.

## Types of Audience

Kimbal Young classified audience into the following types
1. *Information Seeking Audience*—People get together to listen to lectures by well-known people like philosophers, scientists and others. The aim of these people would be to get facts and interpretations and also to make them think and understand the problems.
2. *Conventional Audience*—People get together in large numbers to listen to some religious or political leaders, who have their own ideas and ideologies, which they try to propagate among the people through such meetings. It is a way of influencing the people and trying to convert them to their way of thinking.
3. *Recreational Audience*—Recreational audience is essentially an entertainment seeking audience. For example, a snake-charmer on the road, the circus man, etc. The main aim of all these people is to gather audience and entertain them.

## Influence of Formal and Informal Groups on Health and Sickness

Formal and informal groups are an important aspect of every society. They play an important role in the life of the individual and the society. These groups have an influence on the health and sickness of the people in the society.

Family is a primary informal group that has the greatest impact on the individual. The family has the essential function of bearing and rearing of children. The family members provide for the basic necessities of the individual for his survival. The economic conditions of the family play an important role on the health and sickness of the individuals. The economically better families are able to provide their children with better facilities like education, home, food and other basic necessities when compared to the poorer families. Thus, the poorer families face problems of malnutrition leading to health problems and diseases. Also, they are not able to spend for their treatment of disease and sickness. Lack of education and illiteracy among the poor leads to a lack of awareness among them to prevent health problems, ways to promote health and to cure them. The religious and cultural background of the family also has an impact on the health of the individuals like some superstitions and beliefs may help to improve the health and sometimes may even harm the individual.

The peer group or the friend's circle, which is another important primary, informal group also has an influence on the individual's health. The life style patterns and habits of the individual are greatly influenced by the peer group. For good health, good food habits, healthy recreational activities and games are essential. On the other hand, bad habits like smoking, alcoholism or drug abuse lead to health problems.

The formal or the secondary groups are the groups formed by man to satisfy some of his needs, which are not met within the primary groups. These groups are large in number in the modern complex societies and have a great influence on the individual. The importance of these groups has increased due to the rapid social changes taking place in the society. The hospital, where the child is born today is an example of a formal, secondary group of the society. In the earlier simple society the child was born at home and the family took care of the mother and child. Now the hospital provides the scientific equipments, trained staff, safety and care to the mother and child.

Government and nongovernment organizations also provide a number of services for the individuals like medical camps, blood-donation camps, eye camps, etc. Government also has established a number of primary health centers, general hospitals, etc. to provide health services and for controlling diseases. It also implements a number of health programs to improve the health status of the people. Health education is also given through campaigns and mass media to increase the awareness among the population about health, hygiene and sanitation, health problems, diseases, rehabilitation services for the handicapped, immunization programs, etc. The government is also taking steps to improve the conditions of the industrial workers by providing them with insurance schemes, subsidized lunch, maternity, sickness and medical benefits, which helps in maintaining the health of the worker. It imposes rules on the industries for providing proper conditions of work and safety measures for maintaining the health of the worker.

## The Role of Primary and Secondary Groups in the Hospital and Rehabilitation Set-up

The primary and secondary groups of the society play an important role in the society, as well as in the life of the individual. Both the groups help in fulfilling the needs and helping for the recovery of the patients when hospitalized.

Family is one of the most important primary groups, which satisfies the basic and essential socioeconomic, psychological, and physiological needs of the individual, without which survival would become difficult. In the hospital situation, the family helps the doctor and other staff by providing information about the family history and behavior of the patient, about his needs and sufferings. Such information will be useful for the doctor to treat the patient. Families, in turn, can also take the suggestions from the doctor in taking care of the patient. This will help in the proper care and recovery of the patient.

A patient in the rehabilitation center needs more emotional, social and moral support for now he has to recover from some disability or sickness through intensive education and training. If there is no improvement, the patient has to be educated, mentally and physically, to live with the disability and lead a comfortable life. Here, the role of the family becomes important in providing the moral support to the patient and helping the medical team in preparing the patient to accept the disability or sickness.

Another important primary group is the peer group. It can help the patient, the patient's family and the medical team by providing the necessary emotional, physical and economical support.

The hospital with its medical team is an example of a secondary group, which plays an important role in the patient's life satisfying many of his basic needs like esteem, cognitive, aesthetic and self actualization needs.

The government, another secondary group also tries to help individuals by providing them with money, equipments, buildings and drugs, through government hospitals. This helps especially the poorer sections of people to meet their health needs. It also provides financial assistance to have health schemes and projects. Health education departments of the government hospitals create health awareness about health problems. The government, through its policies, programs and financial aid is able to improve the health of the population.

The government also helps in the rehabilitation of the patients by providing advanced training to medical and paramedical professionals for treatment of patients. It also provides aids to the handicapped and vocational training to suit the handicapped individuals. Voluntary agencies also give support to the patients. They provide self-help services for the patient with selected health problems. Family-centered services are also carried out by voluntary agencies.

Industries play a very important role in the modern man's life. Modern industries provide health insurance schemes for their workers, which gives them maternity benefits, sickness benefits, medical benefits, etc. They also provide financial compensation, pension etc. to the disabled.

### POINTS TO NOTE

1. Definition—Meaning and classification of social groups
2. Types of social groups
    a. Primary and secondary groups
    b. Formal and informal groups
    c. In-groups, out-groups and ethnocentrism
    d. Spatial group–clan or sib–tribe–mob–crowd–public–audience
3. Impact of these groups on health and sickness of individuals.

### NURSING IMPLICATIONS

Man, though born as a biological being becomes a social in the company of other human beings by living in groups, which influence his behvior patterns. A study of these groups therefore helps the nurse to evaluate the patients in a better way.

### QUESTIONS

1. Define:
    a. Social group
    b. Primary and secondary group

c. Formal and informal group
   d. Clan or Sib
   e. Audience
2. What is a crowd? Explain its characteristics.
3. Types of crowd.
4. Meaning of secondary group.
5. Bring out the features of crowd.
6. Characteristics of ingroup.
7. Classification of social groups.
8. Adverse effects of ingroups.
9. Health problems of tribes.
10. Bring out the differences between the following
    a. Primary and Secondary group
    b. Crowd and Audience
    c. Crowd, Public and Audience
11. What is a social group? Describe the characteristics of a primary group.
12. Describe the characteristics of primary and secondary groups.
13. Define a social group. Describe briefly the classification of social groups.
14. Describe the functions of primary and secondary groups.
15. Importance of primary and secondary groups in society.
16. Describe the functions of primary and secondary groups.
17. What is a social group? Describe any two types of social groups.

# CHAPTER 6

# Family and Marriage

**Family**
- Family - functions
- Types – joint, nuclear, blended and extended family: characteristics
- The modern family – changes, problems – dowry, welfare Services, etc.
- Changes and legislations on family and marriage in India-marriage Acts

**Marriage**
- Marriage-forms and functions of marriage
- Marriage and family problems in India
- Family, marriage and their influence on health and health practices

## ■ FAMILY

Family is one of the most basic and important primary groups of the society. The word "family" is derived from the Latin word "famulus" meaning "servant". In Roman Law, the word denoted a group of producers and slaves and other servants, as well as members connected by common descent or marriage. Thus, family meant a group, consisting of a man, a woman, with a child or children and servants.

## Definitions

1. According to Mac Iver, family is "a group defined by sex relationship sufficiently precise and enduring to provide for the procreation and upbringing of children."
2. Eliot and Merril define it as "a biological social unit composed of husband, wife and children."
3. Burgess and Locke define it as "a group of persons united by ties of marriage, blood or adoption, constituting a single household, interacting or intercommunicating with each other in their respective social roles of husband and wife, father and mother, son and daughter, brother and sister, creating common culture."

4. Nimkoff says that "family is a more or less desirable association of husband and wife, with or without a child or of a man or woman alone, with children."

## Characteristics

1. *A Mating Relationship*—A family comes into existence when a man and woman establish a mating relationship between them.
2. *A Form of Marriage*—Mating relationship is established through the institution of marriage. Marriage may take different forms like monogamy, polygamy, polyandry, etc.
3. *Selection of Mates*—There are different ways of selection of mates according to the rules of the society, e.g., it may be done by parents or other elders or the individuals themselves.
4. *A System of Nomenclature and Descent*—Every family has a name. It is known and recognized by this name. The members can trace their descent through the family, which could be either through the male or the female.
5. *A Common Residence*—A family requires a home or a household for its living, bearing and rearing of children.
6. *An Economic Provision*—Family provides for the satisfaction of the economic needs of its members.

## Distinctive Features

Besides the above mentioned general characteristics of the family, there are also certain distinctive characteristics of the family because it has a unique and nuclear position in the social structure of the society. It has a great sociological significance in the society.

1. *Universality*—Family is one of the most important social groups of the society, which is found in all societies, at all times, in the history of man.
2. *Emotional Basis*—Man being a psychological being has certain emotional needs like impulses of mating, procreation and parental care, which can be satisfied in the family. The family is a small, intimate group, which is built upon the sentiments of love, affection, sympathy, cooperation and friendship.
3. *Limited Size*—The size of the family is small. It is limited by the biological conditions.

4. *Formative Influence*—The family has a great formative influence on the individual. It moulds the personality of the individual.
5. *Nuclear Position in the Social Structure*—The family has a nuclear or important position in the social structure of the society. The whole social structure of the society is built of family units.
6. *Responsibility of the Members*—Every member of the family has certain responsibilities, duties and obligations. The family can carry out its functions only when all the members carry out their responsibilities and duties in coordination with each other.
7. *Social Regulation*—The family has its own customs, traditions and legal regulations, which control its members. It is not easy to violate them.
8. *Permanent and Temporary*—Family as an institution is permanent and universal, while, as an association, it is temporary and transitional.

## Functions

Mac Iver classifies the functions of the family as Primary or Essential functions and Secondary or Non-Essential functions.

### *Primary or Essential Functions*

Primary functions of the family are those functions, which are basic for its continued existence.
1. *Stable Satisfaction of Sex Need*—Human beings have a sex instinct. This sex need of man is satisfied through the institution of marriage and family. Thus, it controls and regulates the sexual behavior of man.
2. *Reproduction or Procreation and Rearing of the Children*—The result of sexual satisfaction is procreation or reproduction. Thus, it helps in the perpetuation of the race and propagation of the species. The children that are born are helpless and dependent. The family provides them with the basic necessities for their survival.
3. *Provision of a Home and Affectional Function*—Man being an emotional being, needs care, love and affection from other human beings around him in order to develop as a normal human being. This is satisfied in the family, where he has intimate relationships.

Parents and children are dependent on the home for love and affection, protection and comfort.
4. *An Agent of Socialization*—Family plays a very important role in the socialization of the individual. This process first begins in the family, from the birth of the individual till his death. It shapes the personality of the individual.
5. *An Instrument of Cultural Transmission*—The family teaches the individual the morals, beliefs, values and ideals of the society. It transmits the ideas and ideologies, folkways and mores, customs and traditions, beliefs and values from one generation to another and thus maintains the cultural continuity of the society of which it is a part.
6. *Status Ascribing Function and Social Identification for the Individual*—The family provides the individual with an ascribed status, i.e., a status over which the individual has no choice. His membership in the family is an ascribed status. Also, his ethnic status, religious status, nationality are all ascribed statuses, which are determined by the family. All this gives an identity to the individual in the society.

### *Secondary or Non-Essential Functions*

The family also performs some secondary or non-essential functions for the individual.
1. *Economic Functions*—The traditional family was a self-sufficient unit, fulfilling the economic needs of its members. It was a unit where all the members worked together, producing goods and consuming them. There was a clear cut division of labor between the men and women in the family. Today, this function of the family has changed due to the effects of the process of industrialization and urbanization. The family members work outside the home and are engaged in different kinds of economic activities.
2. *Educational Functions*—The family is an important agency of education for the individual. It is here that the child's basic learning begins. This forms the basis for his adulthood. Today, much of the formal education of the child has been shifted to other formal centers of training like the school, the college and other institutes of learning.

3. *Religious Functions*—The family gives religious training to its children. The child learns the different religious practices, rituals, virtues etc., from its parents in the family. Thus, the religious inheritance is passed on through the family from one generation to another.
4. *Health*—The family takes care of the health of the family members by providing them with basic necessities of life like food, shelter and clothing and taking care of them during the times of sickness or illness. Today, this function is gradually being taken over by hospitals and nurses.
5. *Recreational Functions*—The traditional family was also a center of recreation. All kinds of group activities were arranged, which brought the members together. This increased the solidarity among the members - the old and the young, the women and men of the family. Today, recreational activities take place outside the house—clubs, hotels and theaters, which provide for individual or couple participation. There is no family participation.

## Changes in the Modern Family or Recent Trends in the Modern Nuclear Family

The modern family has been undergoing a number of changes in structure and functions due to the changes taking place in the society. Some of the most important factors bringing about a change in the traditional family are industrialization, urbanization, modernization, democratic ideals, changing status of women and the declining influence of religion, etc. Some of the important changes that can be observed in the institution of family are the following:

1. *Industrialization*—The traditional family was a self-sufficient economic unit—a unit of production, as well as consumption. With the factory system of production, the economic functions of the family are now being performed by the factory. The modern family has now become more of a consumption unit rather than a unit of production.
2. *Urbanization*—Urbanization generally follows industrialization. Urbanization is the growth of towns and cities, which attracts people to migrate. This effects the size of the family. The families are small and the family ties become weak.

3. *Democratic Ideals*—Democratic ideals and principles influence the people. It assures equality and freedom to all, irrespective of sex or creed. Thus, people are able to fulfill their rights and use their power.
4. *Decline of the Influence of Mores and Religious Beliefs*—Religious beliefs, customs, traditions, mores, etc., have become less important for the family. The attitudes and values of the people have changed. Therefore, there is less influence of mores and religious beliefs over the individuals. Religion, which was a form of strong social control in the traditional family is no longer a control over the behavior of the individuals in the family.
5. *Spirit of Individualism and the Development of Romantic Love and Divorce*—Spirit of individualism increases among the people with the principles of democracy influencing them. This has effected the institution of marriage. Marriage toady is based on individual's choice of mate. The authority of the family over the individual is reduced. Marriage has become more of a civil contract rather than a sacred tie between the two individuals. This has also resulted in easy dissolution of marriage or increasing divorce.
6. *Dependence on Outside Agencies for Fulfilling Non-Essential Functions*—Many of the non-essential functions of the family have been taken over by other agencies like educational function taken over by schools, colleges, institutes, or baby sitting, kindergarten, crèches, taking care of children or the hospitals and nurses coming in to help the sick patients. Some economic activities are also performed by agencies like banks, governments.
7. *Economic Independence and Emancipation of Women*—Women working outside the house has given them economic independence. This has resulted in a change in the status of women, enjoying an equal status in all spheres of life with the men in the society.
8. *Decline in the Birth Rate*—With the economic independence and emancipation of women, there is a gradual decline in the birth rate. The families are disintegrating from joint to nuclear.
9. *Parent-youth Conflict*—There is an increasing conflict between the older generation and the younger generation, which is called as the "generation gap".

10. *Filocentric or Pedocentric Family*—The modern family tends to become filocentric. A filocentric family is where the children tend to dominate the scene and their wishes determine the policy of the family. The children decide things for themselves like the college they would like to study in or the kind of food or clothes that they would like to have, etc.

Thus, from the above discussion, the modern family has been undergoing a number of structural and functional changes.

## *Problems of the Modern Family*

It has been observed that the modern family is undergoing a number of changes. This has given rise to a number of problems in the modern family. Some of the major problems are the following.
1. *Lack of Trust and Unity among the Members of the Family*—Most modern families face the problem of lack of trust among its members i.e. between husband and wife, or children and parents, which may also lead to increasing conflicts and disorganization of the family.
2. *Instability*—Many modem families are unstable because marriage is considered more as a contract than a sacred tie between the husband and wife.
3. *Changes in the Relationship of Men and Women*—With the changes in the position of women in the society, there is a change in the relationship of the husband and wife in the family.
4. *Laxity in Marital and Sexual Relationships*—Rigidity associated with sexual relationship in traditional families no longer characterizes the modem family.
5. *Economic Imbalance*—Economic imbalances increase because of the modern style of life and luxurious demands of the family members.
6. *Decline of Religious Controls*—The importance of religion, ideals, values, customs, traditions, is becoming less for the members of modern family. Therefore, there is a decline of controls over the family members, which may lead them to take up to antisocial activities.
7. *Increasing Divorce*—In the modern family, marriage is no longer considered as a sacred bond between the men and the women. It

is more of a legal contract and therefore, there is an increase in the divorce rates.

## Types or Forms of Family

Families have been classified by different sociologists in different ways on the basis of different factors. Some of the important classifications are as follows:

### On the Basis of Marriage

1. *Monogamous Family*—Monogamous family is one in which one man marries only one woman at one time. This is the most common and approved from of family from the biological viewpoint.
2. *Polygamous Family*—Polygamous family is one in which one individual marries more than one individual at one time or on several occasions. Therefore, there are different forms of polygamy.
   a. *Polygyny*—In this form of marriage, one man marries many women and lives as their husband at one time. Polygyny may be:
      i. *Bigamy*—When one man marries two women at the same time.
      ii. *Sororal Polygyny*—When one man marries many women, who are sisters, at the same time.
      iii. *Non-Sororal Polygyny*—When one man marries many women, who are not related, at the same time.
   b. *Polyandry*—In this form of marriage one woman marries many men at the same time and lives as their wife. Polyandry again may be:
      i. *Fraternal Polyandry*—In this, one woman is the wife of many men, who are brothers.
      ii. *Non-Fraternal Polyandry*—In this, one woman is the wife of many men, who are not related to each other.

### On the Basis of Authority or Descent

1. *Patriarchal Family*—The patriarchal family is the most common type of family found in almost all societies. It is a type of family in which the male is the head of family and who has all the authority

and power over all the family matters like administration, property, religious rites of the family, etc. All other members of the family living in it are subordinate to him. Thus, the eldest male member is the protector and ruler of the family, enjoying full powers and authority over the family matters and family members. The important characteristics of the patriarchal family are the following:

a. The father or the eldest male member is the head of the family and therefore, the owner of the family property.
b. Descent is reckoned through the father i.e., the children are known by the name of the family of their father. This is patrilineal.
c. The wife after marriage, comes to live in the home of the husband. This is the patrilocal system.
d. The male children can inherit the property of their father. They have no right over the property of their mother's family. With the passage of the Hindu Code Bill this has undergone a change.

2. *Matriarchal Family*—The matriarchal family is found among some primitive people who lead a wandering or hunting life. In this kind of societies, the male members are away from home for long periods of time, which compelled the women to take care of the family and the home. It is a type of family in which the female is the head of the family and who has all the authority and powers over all the family matters and family members. The male members are subordinate to female members of the family. But in actual practice, even in these families, the male members take up the control of the family. The important characteristics of the matriarchal family are the following:

a. The mother or the eldest female member is the head of the family and the owner of the family property. Therefore, all the authority is in the hands of the wife or some representative of the wife.
b. Descent is reckoned through the mother and not the father because maternity is a fact, while paternity is only an opinion. This is the matrilineal system.

c. Marriage relations are transient. The husband is sometimes merely a casual visitor.
   d. The children are brought up in the home of the wife's relatives. The husband after marriage comes to live in the home of the wife. This is the matrilocal system.
   e. Property is transferred through the mother and only females succeed to it.

## On the Basis of Structure

1. *Nuclear Family*—A nuclear family is the one which consists of the husband, wife and their children. The children leave the parental home as soon as they are married. Therefore, it is an autonomous unit, free from the control of elders.
2. *Joint Family*—The joint family is also known as "undivided family" or an "extended family". This family is made up of a number of nuclear families. It normally consists of members belonging to three generations i.e., husband and wife, with their married and unmarried children and their married and unmarried grand children. It is one of the basic social institutions in the most traditional societies like India. It is controlled by the eldest member of the family.

## On the Basis of Ancestry

1. *Matrilineal Family*—In the Matrilineal family, mother is the basis of ancestry. A woman is believed to be the ancestor of the family. The rights of each member of the family depend on his relation to the mother.
2. *Patrilineal Family* — In the patrilineal family, father is the basis of ancestry. The ancestry continues through the father. This type of family is prevalent today in most societies.

## On the Basis of Residence

1. *Matrilocal Family*—In this type of family, the husband goes to live in the house of his wife after marriage.
2. *Patrilocal Family*—In this type of family, the wife goes and lives in the house of her husband after marriage.

### On the basis of Ingroup and Outgroup Affiliation

1. *Endogamous Family*—An endogamous family is one which sanctions marriage only among members of the ingroup.
2. *Exogamous Family*—An exogamous family sanctions marriage of members of an ingroup with members of an outgroup.

### On the Basis of Blood-Relationships

1. *Conjugal Family*—Conjugal family consists of the spouses, their off springs and relatives through marriage.
2. *Consanguineous Family*—A consanguineous family consists of blood relatives together with their mates and children.

## Indian Family—The Joint Family System

The joint family is also known as the "extended family" or the "undivided family". This type of family was found in the traditional societies like India, and is therefore also known as the "traditional family". The joint family, along with the caste system and the village, played a very important role in the life of the individuals in the Indian society. These are called as the "pillars" on which the whole Hindu society is built.

### Definition

1. I Karve defines a joint family as "a group of people who generally live under one roof, who eat food, cooked at one hearth, who hold property in common and who participate in common family worship and are related to each other as some particular type of kindred."
2. According to I P Desai "a joint family is that household which has greater generation depth than the individual family and the members of which are related to one another by property, income and mutual rights and obligations."

The joint family may be a patriarchal joint family or a matriarchal joint family. The patriarchal joint family is a male-dominated family like the families found among Nambudaris of Malabar or the Nagas of Assam. The matriarchal joint family is a female-dominated family like the families found among the Nairs of Malabar and Khasis and Garos of Assam.

## Characteristics of the Joint Family

The important characteristics of the joint family are the following:
1. *Large in Size*—The joint family consists of parents, children, grand children and other blood relations like uncles, aunts, cousins and others living together. There are at least three or more generations living together.
2. *Common Residence*—The members of the joint family live under the same roof or in a common house.
3. *Common Kitchen*—The members of the joint family have a common kitchen. They eat food cooked at one place. Generally, the eldest female member is in charge of the kitchen.
4. *Common Religion and Worship*—The members of the joint family follow a common religion and worship a common deity. They perform all religious rites and duties and celebrate festivals and social functions jointly. They participate together in all social occasions like marriages, birth, death or any other occasion of happiness or sorrow.
5. *Common Property*—The members of the joint family hold a common property. The head of the family manages the common property. The earnings of all the members are pooled together and used for the family expenses. All those who do not contribute to the property are also supported by this property. They also have a share in the common property.
6. *Exercise of Authority*—The eldest male member has all authority and power over the joint family members and joint family matters in a patriarchal joint family. While in a matriarchal joint family, the eldest female member, in theory, exercises all authority and power over the family. But in practice, it is actually the male members who control the family.
7. *Mutual Rights and Obligations*—All the members of the family identify themselves with the joint family. Each one of the members has his own rights and obligations towards the family. The head of the family alone enjoys certain privileges in the family. He acts as a guide for all the members of the family. The

family in turn protects the interests of its members and takes good care of all of them.
8. *Self-sufficient Unit*—The traditional joint family was a self-sufficient unit. It was a unit of production, as well as consumption. All the needs of the individuals were satisfied within the family itself like economic, recreational, medical, educational, etc.

## Merits and Demerits of the Joint Family System

The joint family system has its own merits and demerits.

### Merits of the Joint Family System

1. *Stable and Durable*—It is more stable and durable than the nuclear family. It is thus able to contribute to the continuation of the cultural traditions. The members may come and go, but the family continues to be there as a social group.
2. *Ensures Economic Progress*—The joint family provides economic security to its members by providing them with the basic necessities of life - food, shelter and clothing - an essential condition of economic progress.
3. *Advantages of Division of Labor*—The work in the joint family is distributed on the principles of division of labor. Every member of the family is given some work according to his ability, like the women and children also work to manage the family matters.
4. *Economy of Expenditure*—There is an economy of expenditure because things are purchased jointly. No single member has an absolute right over the joint property. Also, the head of the family controls the expenditure of the family.
5. *Social Insurance*—The joint family provides the basic necessities of food, shelter, clothing and protection to orphans, widows, deserted, divorced, separated, neglected, sick, old or incapacitated members. It acts as a social insurance.
6. *Social Security*—The joint family also provides social security to its members especially to the weak, aged, sick, infirm, disabled and other needy members.
7. *Provides Leisure*—There is more leisure time for its members because work is shared by all the members and therefore, finish

off the work in less time. This is especially helpful for the women in the family.
8. *Provides Recreation*—The joint family also acts as a place of recreation where all the members come together-the old, the young, the children, the men and the women of the family to spend their leisure time. This increases the bonding between the members of the family.
9. *Social Control*—The joint family acts as a strong agency of social control. The head of the family, with his authority and power, is able to control the behavior of the members. The individual learns to subordinate his interest to that of the family.
10. *Social Virtues*—The joint family is the house of social virtues. The members learn to live in cooperation with each other and develop the qualities of sacrifice, affection, selflessness, broadmindedness, tolerance, loyalty, discipline, generosity, obedience, service-mindedness, etc.

## Demerits of the Joint Family System

1. *Hindrance in the Development of the Individual Personality*—In the joint family, the head of the family, usually the oldest member of the family, has absolute control over all the other members of the family. Thus, individuals do not have the opportunity to become independent or self-dependent. This acts as a hindrance to the development of the personality of the individual. He is not able to develop his talents, qualities of adventure, self-determination, etc. This effects the individuality, creativity and originality of the members.
2. *Promotes Laziness and Idleness*—The joint family provides social and economic security to all its members. They are assured of the basic necessities of life. Therefore, many of them do not do any work. In most joint family, some people toil, while some lead a life of lethargy.
3. *Not Favorable for Savings and Investments*—Individual savings and investment habits are not encouraged because they have to share their income with the other family members. Also, individuals do not feel the need to save as they are taken care of by the joint family.

4. *Center of Quarrels*—The joint family is the house of quarrels and problems of adjustments and misunderstandings among the members. There are constant quarrels especially among the women folk and the old and the young.
5. *Encourages Litigation*—The joint family members resort to law especially at the time of the division of the common property.
6. *Lack of Privacy*—There is a lack of privacy for the individuals in the joint family especially for the newly wedded couples. Due to the presence of a number of members in the family, they rarely get an opportunity to come close to each other and get an opportunity to talk about their personal matters. Hence, they do not develop any intimacy.
7. *Adverse Effect on Socialization of Children*—The socialization of the children in the joint family is affected. The parents cannot give their personal attention to their children. The children are under the control and care of the older people in the family. They become more attached to them. The parents are not given the opportunity to bring up their children in the way they want. They have to be brought up according to the old traditions and customs of the family.
8. *Low Status of Women*—In the traditional joint families, which were mostly patriarchal, the position of the women was very low. She was all the time, through out her life, under the control of the male members. She did not have any freedom in the family. This lead to a lot of frustration and depression among the women.
9. *Uncontrolled Reproduction*—In a joint family the married members do not feel the necessity to restrict the number of children. This is because, the children are taken care of by the family. The basic needs and necessities are provided by the family and therefore, the parents do not feel the burden or responsibility of bringing-up their children.
10. *Limits Social Mobility*—The joint family is very traditional and therefore does not allow any change to take place. It does not accept any modern trends. Social mobility therefore gets restricted.

### Disintegration of the Joint Family System

The Indian society has experienced a number of social changes in the last few years. The traditional institutions of joint family, marriage, caste and village have been effected by these social changes in the society. They have affected the traditional structure, function and stability of these institutions. Some of the important factors, responsible for bringing about social change and thereby effecting a change and disintegration of the traditional joint family system are the following:

1. *Education*—Modern education was introduced in India by the British government. Their system of education was based on their democratic principles and ideologies, i.e. education for all irrespective of any differences. The content of education imparted also was based on democratic ideas and ideologies. This influenced the Indians, especially the younger generations. It brought about a change among them, in their attitudes, values, beliefs, ideals, etc. towards the traditional institutions like the family and marriage, caste, etc. As the educational levels increase, job opportunities also increase and economic independence increases. All these factors effect the relationships among the members of the joint family. With their new ideas and ideologies gained through education, they no longer like to live in a joint family. They set-up their own individual families.

2. *Industrialization*—Industrialization is the growth of factory system of production. This creates employment opportunities, which attract people of the rural areas. The people in rural areas are dependent on agriculture. The joint family system is suitable for this agricultural occupation. But, with the increase in population, all the population do not have jobs on the land. Therefore, the people start moving to the industrial centers, which breaks down the joint family of the village. Industrialization also effects the traditional small scale industries. Their products cannot compete with the products produced in the large scale factory system of production. Gradually, they have to close down their production due to losses. With this closing down of their industries, the villagers are compelled to move to the industrial centers, where there are employment opportunities. Thus, the joint family system disintegrates.

3. *Urbanization*—Urbanization is the phenomenon of the growth of towns and cities. Urban centers are more developed than the villages in terms of facilities like education of children, hospitals, entertainment, recreation, employment opportunities, etc.

Therefore, they become centers of attraction especially for the rural population. Thus, there is a movement of the rural population from the village to the urban areas. This effects a breakup of the joint family system in the village. Besides this, the urban pattern of living is not suitable for living in a joint family. Thus, the nuclear family emerges in urban areas.

4. *Western Influence*—India has a great influence of the west, with the democratic system of education introduced by the British in their schools in India. The educated youth took up to these democratic principles of equality, freedom, rationalism, individualism, etc. These ideas went against the joint family and gradually brought about a disintegration of the joint family.

5. *Social Legislation*—A number of new laws regarding marriage and family have effected the joint family system. They have brought about a change in the relations among the family members, the composition and the stability of the joint family system. Some of the important social legislations effecting marriage and family in India are the Child Marriage Restraint Act, 1929 and the Hindu Marriage Act, 1955, fixed the minimum age of marriage for the boys and girls and to marry according to their wishes. The Special Marriage Act, 1954 gave the freedom of mate selection and marriage to the individual. These laws effected the role of the elders' authority in deciding the marriage of the children in the family. The Widow Remarriage Act, 1856 — gives sanction for widow remarriage, The Hindu Marriage Act, 1955 — permits divorce and the Hindu Succession Act, 1956 - gives a share to the daughters in parental property. All these acts have effected solidarity of the joint family system and the relationships among its members

From the above discussion, it appears that the joint family is gradually breaking up and the nuclear family is taking its place. From various studies conducted in the Indian villages by scholars like KM Kapadia, Dr I Karve, Aileen D Ross, IP Desai, MS Gore and others, show that though there is a disintegration of the joint family system in India, but at a very slow pace. The joint family continues to be an important institution in the Indian villages but with a difference. The modern joint family has undergone a change in its structure like it may be smaller in size compared to the traditional family. There are also corresponding changes in its functions, some of which have been taken over by specialized agencies like the schools, hospitals, etc. This is because the village and the agricultural occupation are suitable for the continuation of the joint family. Also, it is observed that those individuals who migrate away from the villages to the urban-industrial centers for various reasons continue to maintain their relationship with joint family. This can be noticed in their frequent visits to their village, especially for all important occasions like marriage, festivals, ceremonies, etc. Even the educated modern youth feel, it is their moral obligation and duty to maintain their relationship with the parent joint family. Thus, though physically they may be staying away from the joint family, sentimentally and emotionally, they are still attached to it and continue to maintain their ties with the joint family. This shows that the joint family has not completely died out though it may be disintegrating.

## Nuclear Family or Modern Family

The modern nuclear family is a universal phenomenon in almost all the societies today. It consists of the husband, wife and unmarried children. After marriage, the children set up their own separate household. Thus, it is more autonomous and independent, free from the control of the elders. It is a characteristic of modern urban-industrial centers and more suitable for the modern societies. It continues to perform the sexual, the reproductive, the economic and the educational functions.

### *Structure of the Nuclear Family*

The nuclear family consists of only the husband, the wife and the unmarried children. Thus, it consists of only two generations. There are restrictions of marriage among the members of the family. Therefore, a third generation can be formed only by the exchange of males and females between the existing families. This gives rise to two kinds of nuclear families:
1. The family of orientation in which the individual is born and brought-up and which includes the father, the mother, brothers and sisters.
2. The family of procreation, which the individual establishes by his marriages and which includes the husband, the wife, the sons and the daughters.

### Features of the Nuclear Family

Some of the important features of the modern nuclear family are the following:

1. *Choice of Mates*—In the traditional family, the selection of marriage partners was done by the elder members of the family. In the modern family, there is less parental control and interference. The individual selects his own mate either with or without the consent of parents. It is more of an individual and personal choice.
2. *Changes in the Relationship of the Man and the Woman*—The man and the woman have an equal status in the modern family. She is equally educated, emancipated and empowered today. She exercises her authority and power equally like the man in the family. She is no longer subservient to him like in the patriarchal joint family.
3. *Laxity in Sex Relationships*—Illegitimate sex relationships of the husband and wife are on the increase in the modern family.
4. *Economic Independence*—Equal opportunities of education and working outside the home of the women has emancipated them and made them economically independent. This has effected the attitude of the women towards the man and towards the number of children in the family. She no longer feels obliged to stay under the control of the male members, be it her husband or children.
5. *Decline of the Traditional Controls of the Customs, Traditions, Beliefs, Religion, etc.*—The traditional social controls of customs, traditions, beliefs, religion, etc., are loosing their importance for the members of the modern family. Marriage is also considered to be a civil contract and not a religious sacrament. Therefore, the control of religion over marriage has become less. Divorce has become a common phenomenon in the family.
6. *Filocentric or Pedocentric Family*—The modern family is tending to become filocentric in nature. A filocentric family is one in which the children tend to dominate the family and their wishes become important for the family. They determine the policy of the family. Physical punishment is not given to the children. The children decide their personal aspects of their life like the kind of school or college they would like to go to, the course they want to study, the kind of clothes they want to wear, the kind of food that they would like to eat etc.

7. *Separation of Non-Essential Functions*—Many of the traditional functions of the family have been given up by the modern family. They have been taken over by specialized agencies in the society like the school, the hospitals, the hotels, clubs, old age homes, kindergartens, etc.

Thus, from the above discussion, it can be said that the traditional Indian family has undergone a number of economic, social and biological changes. It is no longer a self-sufficient unit of the traditional society. There is a change in the size, structure and functions of the family. The modern family is more individualized and democratic. Burgess therefore referred to the modern family as "a unity of interacting personalities."

## Family Welfare Services

Family is one of the most important and basic primary groups of the society. It provides the social and psychological security to the individual. It takes care of the health of its members by providing them with the basic necessities of life. The socialization of the individual begins in the family and is responsible for the development of the personality of the individual.

India is one of the first countries in the world to adopt the Family Planning Program in 1952, which was later changed to "Family Welfare", which is voluntary. The main aim of this policy is to promote family welfare, to provide comprehensive health services like maternal, child health and family planning services and to improve the standard of living.

Family welfare services include sex education, advice on sterility, planned parenthood, counseling, premarital consultation and examination, marriage counseling, spacing and limitation of births, screening for pathological conditions related to the reproductive tract infections, home economics, services for unmarried mothers, safe water supply, control and prevention of communicable diseases, safe disposal of excreta, providing of adoption services, promoting women and child health, reproductive and child health (RCH) program activities, to raise the living standards of people, measures to improve educational facilities, compulsory education for children, conducting information education communication(IEC) campaigns to change the deep rooted beliefs, attitudes and practices related to large family size, raising the age of marriage, improving the status of women and old age security.

## MARRIAGE

- Marriage-Forms and Functions of Marriage
- Marriage and Family Problems in India
- Family, Marriage and their influence on health and health practices.

Marriage is one of the most important social institutions of the society. It plays a very important role in the life of the individual, as well as the society. In most societies, it is considered as religious, besides providing a basis for the family and the satisfaction of sexual urges of man. It has been established in the human society to control and regulate the sex life of man. According to Bogardus, marriage is an institution for admitting men and women to a family.

### Definitions

1. Gillin and Gillin define marriage as "a socially approved way of establishing a family of procreation."
2. According to Edward Westermark marriage is "the more or less durable connection between the male and the female, lasting beyond the mere act of propagation till after the birth of the offspring."
3. Malinowski defined marriage as "a contract for the production and maintenance of children."
4. Horton and Hunt say that "marriage is the approved social pattern, whereby two or more persons establish a family."
5. According to Robert H. Lowie "marriage is a relatively permanent bond between permissible mates."
6. DN Majumdar defines marriage as "a socially sanctioned union of a male and female for purposes of establishing a household, entering into sex relations, procreating and providing care for the offsprings."

### Forms of Marriage

The main forms of marriage are the following:
1. *Monogamy*—Monogamy is the most common and universal form of marriage among most people in the society. It is a form of marriage in which one man marries one woman only at one

time. It is the most approved and ideal form of marriage from the biological point of view. According to Malinowski "monogamy is, has been and will remain the only true type of marriage" in any society.

2. *Polygamy*—Polygamy is that form of marriage in which one individual marries more than one individual at one time or on several occasions. Therefore, there are different types of polygamy.
   i. *Polygyny*—In this form of marriage, one man marries more than one women and lives as their husband at one time. Polygyny again may be:
      a. *Bigamy*—When one man marries two women at the same time.
      b. *Sororal Polygyny*—Is that type of marriage in which one man marries many women at the same time. These women are invariably sisters.
      c. *Non-sororal Polygyny*—Is that type of marriage in which one man marries many women at the same time. These women are not related to each other.
      d. *Group Marriage*—Is the marriage of two or more women with two or more men at the same time. The sexual relationships among them are not defined clearly. The children born of such relationships are regarded as the children of the whole group. This kind of a marriage is practically not existing today.
   ii. *Polyandry*—In this form of marriage, one woman marries many men, at the same time and lives as their wife. Polyandry again may be:
      a. *Fraternal Polyandry*—In this form of marriage, one woman is the wife of many men, who are brothers.
      b. *Non-Fraternal Polyandry*—In this form of marriage, one woman is the wife of many men, who are not related to each other. Polyandry is gradually disappearing even from those societies in which it was practiced.

3. *Endogamy and Exogamy*—Endogamy and Exogamy are the rules or restrictions of selection of mates in marriage in any society.
   *Endogamy*—Endogamy is the rule of marriage that one must marry within one's own group. For e.g., it could be tribal endogamy, caste endogamy, subcaste endogamy, class endogamy, race endogamy, etc.

*Exogamy*—Exogamy is the rule of marriage in which one must marry outside his own group. It prohibits marriage within the group. It is the opposite of endogamy. This rule of marriage states that close blood-relations or near relations are not supposed to marry among themselves. There are different forms of exogamy found in India like gotra exogamy, pravara exogamy, village exogamy and pinda exogamy.

4. *Intercaste Marriages*—According to caste rules, intercaste marriages are not allowed among the Hindus. Intercaste marriage means the union of a man and woman belonging to two different castes. But two types of intercaste marriages have been accepted by the Hindus since ancient times.
   a. *Anuloma*—In this type of marriage, a man belonging to the higher caste marries a women belonging to the lower caste.
   b. *Pratiloma*—In this type of marriage, a man belonging to the lower caste marries a woman belonging to the higher caste.

   The rejection and prevention of intercaste marriages is based upon the notions of purity and cultural differences between the various castes. But these differences between the different castes are gradually decreasing due to the influence of western culture.

5. *Hypergamy*—In this type of marriage, the parents wanted to marry their daughters into noble families, which had a very important place in the society. This practice prevailed in Bengal.

6. *Child Marriage*—Child marriage is the practice of the marriages of children. It is performed before the attainment of puberty of the men and the woman.

## Marriage and Family Problems in India

Marriage and family problems in India are due to certain conditions prevalent in the society. They are the following:

1. *Lower Status of Women*—The status of the Indian women has always been lower than that of the men in the society. The Indian family is mostly patriarchal and therefore, the woman is under the control of the man in the family. She does not have any social, economic, political and religious independence. Also, some of the social practices like the practice of sati, child marriages, restrictions of widow remarriage, further lowered her position

in the society. She was not given an opportunity and freedom to develop her individuality and personality.
2. *Reform Movement*—Social reformers like Raja Ram Mohan Roy, Ishwarchandra Vidyasagar, Justice Ranade, Mahatma Gandhi and others tried to bring about changes in the society with the help of social legislation and education. It helped to put an end to some of the evil and inhuman practice in the society. This also helped to improve the position of the women in the society.
3. *Dowry System*—One of the evil practices of marriage in Indian society is the dowry system. Dowry system started as a custom of giving gifts to the daughter from the parents at the time of marriage. It is the money, property or valuables, which the bride's party has to give to the groom's party at the time of marriage. But gradually it has become a social evil. Toady, the bride's party is compelled to give it in exchange of marriage, failing which, the bride has to suffer the consequences at the hands of her in laws, including the husband, in many cases. The government of India has legally banned this practice but it continues to be practiced in the society.

## Legislation of Indian Marriage and Family

The traditional Hindu marriage and the joint family had a number of defects and customs, which were affecting, especially the women in the society. Therefore, social reformers tried to bring about changes in the system. Also, during the British rule and after Independence, legislations were passed to bring about changes in the traditional patterns of family and marriage in India. Some of the most important legislation effecting changes in the Hindu marriage and family and the status of women in India are the following:

1. *Hindu Married Women's Rights to Separate Residence and Maintenance Act 1946*—According to this act, the Hindu married women can claim maintenance while residing separate from the husband under specific conditions.
2. *Hindu Marriage Act 1955*—This act applies to all the members of the Hindu society. It has affected important changes in the Hindu Marriage like classification of Hindu marriages, determination of age of marriage for both the boys and girls, provision of monogamy,

provision for the guardianship of the mother, provision for divorce, etc.

3. *Hindu Succession Act 1956*—According to this act, the daughter also has an equal right of inheritance in the property of the father, along with the son.
4. *Hindu Adoption and Maintenance Act 1956*—According to this act the husband has to take the consent of the wife while adopting a son or daughter and the issueless widow also gets the rights of adoption under specific conditions.
5. *Hindu Minority and Guardianship Act 1956*—This act provides for the guardianship of child, unmarried daughter and illegitimate son and the married daughter.
6. *The Child Marriage Restraint Act 1929*—This act restrains the marriage of a child. According to this act marriage of boys under 21 years of age and girls under 18 years of age is an offence.
7. *Special Marriage Act of 1954*—According to this act, Hindu marriage is a "civil marriage" and provided legal permission for intercaste, interreligious and even registered marriages.
8. *The Hindu Widow Remarriage Act 1856*—This act gives legal sanction for widow remarriage.

## Influence of Family on the Individual's Health

### Family and Nutrition

Family is the most important primary group in the individual's life, taking care of him from his birth till his death. It has the functions of bearing and rearing the child for its survival in the society. It has to take care of the child by providing it with the basic necessities of food, shelter and clothing for its survival. Thus, the family has an influence on the individual's health. Health of the individual is related to the nutrition that he gets.

Nutrition may be defined as the science of food and its relation to health. It is concerned with the part played by "nutrients" or "food" in the growth, development and maintenance of the body. The word "nutrient" is used for specific dietary constituents, such as proteins, vitamins and minerals. Good nutrition helps the individual to grow well and enjoy good health. Food has been recognized as an important factor in the individual's health and disease status. Nutrition is associated with infection, immunity, fertility, maternal and child health and family health.

In recent years, it has been recognized that nutrition is not only a medical problem but a multifactorial problem like socio-economic development. Improvement in health and nutrition can be brought about by solving the problem of poverty, unemployment and injustice. It is an accepted fact that the nutritional problems can be solved by a broad integrated approach of sectors of development.

Family plays an important role in determining the nutritional status of the individual.

1. The economic status of the family determines the kind of nutrition, it is able to provide for its members. For example, economically poor families are not able to provide good nutritious food for its members, which may result in malnutrition.
2. The cultural factor also has its impact on the pattern of food consumption in the family. Some communities may be restricting their food due to this factor like vegetarianism or non-vegetarianism, which may again cause some deficiencies and problems of health.
3. The educational and occupational levels of the family have an influence on the diet of the individuals. These factors increase the awareness about nutrition and health among them and therefore, they take a well planned and balanced diet.
4. Gender differentiation, especially among the patriarchal families leads to problems of malnutrition among the female members.

## *Effects of Sickness in the Family*

Sickness or illness among the members of the family causes disturbances in the family like economic and psychological disturbances. The greatest impact of sickness in the family is the financial burden on the members. This becomes a greater problem, if the afflicted individual is the earning member of the family with a number of dependents. He may not be able to work and contribute towards the family income. On the other hand, family expenditures may increase for the medical treatment of the individual.

Family and Marriage

With a sick person in the family, the routine activities of the other members get distributed. The family relationships and family leisure get affected. The role functioning of the members may also get affected due to sickness in the family, which may lead to emotional disturbances also. In general, all the members of the family, including the children will be affected physically, as well as psychologically by the sickness in the family.

Family therefore plays an important role both in health and sickness or disease of individual. For example, the prevention and treatment of individual illness, the care of dependent adults and children and the stabilization of the personality of both adults and children.

### POINTS TO NOTE
1. Definition–meaning–functions and changes in the types of family and marriage.
2. Legislation and problems of marriage and family.
3. Types:
    a. Traditional Indian joint family and the modern nuclear family
    b. Monogamy and polygamy
    c. Patriarchal and matriarchal
    d. Endogamous and exogamous
    e. Conjugal and consanguineous
4. Influence of family and marriage on the individuals health and health practices, nutrition and sickness in the family.

### NURSING IMPLICATIONS
Family and marriage are the most basic and important social groups of the society to which man belongs. His basic or primary socialization takes place which effects his behavior patterns. The health of the individual is affected by his economic, social and psychological background. Knowledge of all these is clear from the study of his family and marriage patterns.

### QUESTIONS
1. Aims of marriage.
2. Disintegrating factors of joint family.
3. Define dowry.
4. What is fraternal polyandry?

5. What are the provisions of the Hindu Marriage Act?
6. What are the benefits of the Hindu Succession Act for the women?
7. Sorroral polygyny.
8. Define marriage and family.
9. Functions of the family.
10. Benefits of the joint family.
11. What are the adverse health effects of child marriage?
12. Give a brief account of the features of the family and different types of family.
13. Distinguish between the joint family and the nuclear family.
14. Marriage and family problems in India.
15. Define marriage and explain its types.
16. Explain the legislations on Indian marriage and family.
17. Describe changes in the functions of the family in modern India.
18. Describe the changing trends in the modern family and its impact on health and diseases.
19. Explain the advantages and disadvantages of the joint family system.
20. Discuss the major causes of family disorganization.

# CHAPTER 7

# Rural Community

> Features of village community
> Characteristics of Indian village
> Change in Indian rural life
> Problems of villages
> Rural health problems
> Urban health problems
> Community development project and planning

Man is a social animal. He cannot live alone. He gets into relationships with other human beings, who form a group. Community is an organized social group of a locality. According to MacIver, it is "an area of social living marked by some degree of social coherence". He also adds that "whenever the members of any group, small or large, live together in such a way that they share, not this or that particular interest, but the basic conditions of a common life, we call that group a community". When people continue to live in the same locality for a very long time, they tend to develop an attachment and sentimental identification with the area in which they live. This gives rise to a "we feeling" among the people.

Communities are generally classified as tribal, rural and urban. This classification is more or less universally accepted. It is based on the size and density of the population.

## ■ THE RURAL OR VILLAGE COMMUNITY

The word "rural" is derived from the Latin word "ruralis" meaning "a village" or "a town" or "a country". The rural society is many times referred to as an "agrarian society" because the main occupation of the people is agriculture. In the development of human communities, rural community has preceded urban life. The village is the oldest human community.

A rural community consists of people living in a limited physical area, who have common interests and ways in dealing and satisfying them. In spite of the growth of cities, the rural community continues to be important for the society. A major portion of the world population lives in villages and the urban communities are dependent on them even today.

## Definition

1. According to J.H. Kolb and Brunner, a rural community is "a group of people, permanently residing in a definite geographic area, who having developed a certain community consciousness and cultural, social and economic relations, feel that they are separate from other communities."
2. Dwight Sanderson defined a rural community as "people, who are staying together and living on dispersed farmsteads and in a hamlet or village, which forms the center of their common activities."

## Features of the Village Community

Some of the important features or characteristics of the village or rural communities are the following:

1. *Agricultural Occupation*—The main occupation of the rural community is agriculture and some small-scale activities and crafts like pottery, basket-making, spinning and weaving, carpentry, animal husbandry, poultry, bee-keeping, fishing, etc. Therefore, there is less specialization and division of labor in the rural community.
2. *Natural Environment*—The rural people live in a natural environment, with animals, birds, rivers, ponds and other natural things around them. They have a simple and natural life style.
3. *Small Size*—The rural communities are small in size i.e. the number of houses, as well as the number of people living in it is few.
4. *Low Density of Population*—The density of population in rural areas is low, because the number of people inhabiting it is few.
5. *Homogeneity*—The rural community is homogenous. There is unity and uniformity in their social life. They have a common occupation and a common way of life. The community has the same customs, traditions and values.

6. *Low Mobility*—There is very low physical, as well as social mobility in rural areas. Physical mobility is low due to the lack of transport and communication facilities. Social mobility is also low due to certain social conditions, which restrict the movement of the people.
7. *Less Social Differentiation and Stratification*—The rural community being homogenous, there is less social differentiation and stratification.
8. *Primary Group Relations*—The rural communities are small in size. Therefore, the people have personal, informal and intimate relationships. They maintain regular contact with each other.
9. *Large Family*—The rural family is mostly a joint family, suited for the agricultural occupation. It is one of the most important institutions of the village, since the rural community is built around it.
10. *Conservatism, Religion, Customs, Traditions and Social Change*—Conservatism, religion, customs and traditions play a very important role in the life of the people. They act as strong social controls over the individuals. Their beliefs in their religion, customs and traditions, make them conservative. They do not accept any social change very easily.

## ■ CHARACTERISTICS OF THE INDIAN VILLAGE

The Indian village has certain peculiar characteristics, which makes it distinct from other villages. This is because of the institution of caste and joint family in the village, which plays a very important role in social, economic and political organization of the village. Therefore, the village has a very important place in the Indian social structure. India is also called as a land of villages, since major portion of its population live in the villages.

The main occupation of the rural population in India is agriculture along with some cottage industries. They live a life of simplicity in natural conditions or environment. The population is homogenous, living as a small community and therefore having very intimate relationships with each other. Some of the important characteristics of the Indian village are the following:

1. *Self-Sufficiency*—The traditional typical Indian villages were self-sufficient units. They were units of production, as well as

consumption. All their economic and social necessities were satisfied in the village itself. They were isolated or cutoff from the rest of the world outside the village.

2. *Primary Institution*—The Indian village is like a primary institution. It is like a large joint family, where the members have very close and intimate relationships with each other. It plays a very important role in the life of the people and also has an important place in the social structure of the Indian society. The villages are known as one of the pillars of the Indian society along with the joint family and the caste system.

3. *Religious Outlook*—The people of the village are highly religious. They are nature worshippers because of their dependence on nature for their agricultural occupation. It plays a very important role in the life of the people and acts as a strong social control.

4. *Conservatism*—Belief in religion being an important aspect of Indian rural life, customs and traditions play an important role in their life. Therefore, they are conservative and not like to change or accept changes very easily.

5. *Importance of the Family System and other Primary Institutions*—The primary institutions like the joint family and the caste system play a very important role in rural India. They dominate and control the different aspects of the individual's life.

6. *Local self-Government*—The traditional Indian villages had their own governing body called the Panchayats or the Caste Panchayats of the ancient times. They were autonomous political bodies, which managed the village affairs.

7. *Poverty and Illiteracy*—Poverty and illiteracy of the people in Indian villages are common features. Agriculture being the only occupation and with the population pressure increasing on the land, with less employment opportunities, the people are poor. Illiteracy is also high because of their poverty and lack of educational facilities in the village.

8. *Group Feeling and Importance of Neighborhood*—Group feeling and neighborhood are of great importance in Indian villages. They develop very close and intimate relationships with the people in their area. Leading a collective life, sharing the joys and sorrows together, they participate in all activities and matters of the village.

9. *Free from the Problems of Urban Life*—There are less social problems in rural areas. They lead a simple life, with simple needs. Their values and moral standards are high. They also have strong informal social controls like their religion, beliefs, customs, traditions, values, family, caste, etc., which control their behavior patterns. Therefore, they are free from the problems of urban living.
10. *Caste and Social Mobility*—Caste is a form of social stratification, which is a peculiar feature of the Indian village. It is a hierarchical division of the society, a very rigid and closed system, which does not allow any kind of intermixing or social relationship among the different caste groups. This leads to a lack of social mobility in the village.

## ■ CHANGE IN INDIAN RURAL LIFE

Change is a law of nature. The village community also undergoes change though the speed of change may be slow. Many of the characteristic features of the traditional Indian village are also changing. The development of science and technology, the processes of industrialization, urbanization, modernization, westernization, universalization of education, modern medicine, transportation and communication etc., have effected a change in the traditional Indian village.

### Factors of Change

Some of the major factors bringing about change in the Indian rural life are the following:

1. *Natural Factors*—The natural factors of change are those natural elements found in a particular geographical area. They include factors like rain, rivers, floods, storms, draught, earth quakes, mountains, vegetation, animals, etc. They influence changes in the rural community. These factors of nature cannot be controlled by man and therefore he has to adjust himself to the changing conditions in the environment around him. Change therefore takes the form of adaptation.
2. *Technological Factors*—Technological factors include all the new application of science and knowledge. These changes have an

effect on man's life. For example, the availability of electricity to the village, transforms the rural community

3. *Social Factors*—Social factors have an effect on the social life of the rural community. The major social factors affecting rural India are the caste system, the joint family system, marriage, social and religious customs and traditions, etc. A change in any one of the factors effects a change in the rural community. For example, the hold of caste on the village becomes less important with the changes in the caste occupations effected by industrialization. Changes can also be observed in the "jajmani" system, a peculiar feature of the village community in India. The joint family system is being replaced by the nuclear family system, where the individuals have more independence. Change can also be observed in the marriage patterns like the practice of sati and child marriages gradually getting reduced. The standard of living of the village community is going higher with the impact of industrialization, urbanization, modernization and improvements in transport and communication.

4. *Economic Factors*—The economic factors are those which effect their agricultural occupation, trade and business and their small scale cottage industries. With the increase in population, the pressure on the land increases and the problems of unemployment and poverty arise in the rural areas. On the other hand, industrialization and urbanization attract the rural population, due to which they migrate to these areas for various reasons. Improvement in transport and communication also make it easier for them to migrate. All these factors affect the economic conditions in the rural community and bring about changes in the community.

5. *Cultural Factors*—Cultural factors include the beliefs, values, attitudes, customs, traditions, etc. Changes in these aspects of culture bring about changes in the rural institutions like marriage, family, caste, etc.

6. *Political Factors*—Political changes effect the village community. Today, there is greater political consciousness and participation among the rural people because of the spread of education and improvements in transport and communication. Also, change is being effected by planned efforts of the government.

The above mentioned factors are responsible for bringing about a change in the Indian rural community. Change is taking place though at a slow rate. More efforts have to be made to bring about changes in the rural community, so that the differences between the rural and urban communities can be minimized and many of the problems, for both the rural and urban communities can be reduced.

Some of the major changes taking place in rural India are the following:

1. *Changes in Rural Marriage and Family*—There are changes in rural marriage and family like the practice of widow remarriage or the abolition of practices of sati and child marriage to a certain extent. The joint family system is gradually changing to the nuclear family system, resulting in a change in the authority of the family and the status of the women in the family.
2. *Changes in Economic Life*—The traditional occupational pattern of caste is changing. Modern scientific methods are used in agriculture. Modern methods of transport and communication, the electrification of the villages, etc., have effected a change in their business and trade. The very life style of the people has changed.
3. *Changes in Social Life*—Some of the social factors like caste, marriage and family are losing their importance for the individuals in the village. They no longer have a strong hold on them. Educational facilities have improved and the rate of literacy is increasing. There is greater intermixing and interaction between the different caste groups. Governmental intervention is also improving the socio economic conditions of the village community.
4. *Changes in Political Life*—There is great political consciousness and political participation in the villages. Rural leadership (both men and women) is becoming more important. Also villagers are becoming aware of party-based elections.

## ■ COMMUNITY DEVELOPMENT PROJECT AND PLANNING

The Community Development Program (CDP) aims at a comprehensive and all-round development of the village community and the rural people. It is to improve the social economic and cultural conditions of the whole community with the active participation of the government, as well as the community. It is a program, based on philosophy of a program of the people, by the people and for the people. The idea is to integrate the community with the nation.

The government of India established the Planning Commission in March 1950. This commission laid down the CDP on October 2, 1952. The CDP is a part of the Five Year Plans of India. The aim of the Five Year Plans is to bring about an all-round development of the country in a planned way, where as the community development program is for the village community. The planning commission of the government of India has defined it as "an attempt to bring about a social and economic transformation of the village life through the efforts of the people themselves".

Aims—The main aims of the community development program are the following:

1. Integrated development of the social, economic and cultural aspects of the rural community.
2. Development of the available human and material resources.
3. Develop a sense of initiative, awareness and responsibility among the rural people.
4. Develop agriculture, cottage industries and animal husbandry.
5. Improvement of transport, communication, health, sanitation, housing, education and women and child welfare.

## ▓ PROBLEMS OF VILLAGES OR RURAL COMMUNITY

The rural community or the villages have a number of problems due to the changes taking place in the society. Factors like industrialization, urbanization, modernization, westernization and the improvements in transport and communication have effected the self-sufficiency of the villages.

1. There is an opposition to social change. They will not accept changes very easily. This is due to their low educational levels and ignorance. They follow the old practices of cultivation and are also dependent on nature, which results in poor yields.
2. The rate of growth of population in rural India is very high. Therefore, there is a problem of unemployment, which leads to a heavy pressure on the land due to sub-division and fragmentation

of the land holdings. They are also steeped in poverty and the burden of loans.
3. Migration of the landless laborers to urban areas is increasing due to the lack of opportunities in the villages and also to escape from the exploitation by money lenders, officials and rich farmers.
4. There is a lack of civic amenities like transport and communication, medical facilities, educational facilities, water and electricity, etc.
5. The villagers are traditional and illiterate. They are controlled by customs, traditions and superstitions, etc.
6. Due to illiteracy, ignorance and poverty, the rural people are also taking up to evil habits and practices like smoking, alcoholism, gambling, prostitution, etc., and the social problems are increasing.

## Rural Health Problems

The rural communities suffer from a number of health problems, which arise due to their ignorance and illiteracy, coupled with the lack of basic amenities like medical facilities, hospitals, nursing homes, maternity homes, drug shops, clinics and clinical laboratories. The problems of overpopulation, unemployment and poverty, makes it difficult for them to have basic necessities of life like good nutritious food, shelter and clothing. In times of illness or diseases, the people still follow traditional methods like going to a place of worship or for witchcraft to cure their diseases. Added to these problems are the lack of sanitation and the medical personnel hesitating to go to work in rural areas.

Today, the health care professionals and the rural administrative bodies are giving importance to rural health. Voluntary organizations have also taken up the cause of rural welfare. With the improvement in rural education, the rural people have realized the importance of modern medical facilities to maintain their health. Rural welfare activities are an important means of bringing about progress of the rural community. Some of the rural welfare activities are rural education, rural economic development, provision of civic amenities, welfare of the children, women, unemployed persons, agricultural laborers and the weaker sections of the village.

# Rural Community

## POINTS TO NOTE
1. Features of the rural community.
2. Characteristics of the Indian village.
3. Factors of change in the Indian rural life.
4. Problems of rural life and rural health problems.
5. Community development projects (CDP) and planning.

## NURSING IMPLICATIONS
The study of the rural community helps the nurse to understand the background of the patients, especially in the Indian conditions where the major population lives. The study of the rural living conditions gives an insight into their health problems.

## QUESTIONS
1. Define:
    a. Indian rural community
    b. Social welfare
    c. Rural society
    d. Rural development
    e. Community development
2. Features of Indian villages.
3. Problems of rural community.
4. Health problems of rural community.
5. Describe briefly the characteristics or features of rural community.
6. Explain the impact of the community development programs on Indian villages.

# CHAPTER 8
# Urban and Regional Community

- Urban—the growth in the cities
- Features of urban community
- City community in India
- Urban-rural contrast
- Major urban problems
- The Regional community

## ■ URBAN—THE GROWTH IN THE CITIES

The term "urban" means "city". It is generally used to denote a "civilized" society. The history of every civilization is the history of its towns and cities. "Civilization" means "the city" and "the city" means "civilization". Civilization is the product of man and his achievements. Therefore, it is said that man built the city and the city in turn civilized man.

The history of the growth of cities can be traced back to 6000 BC and 5000 BC. These could not be called as cities in their true sense. They were small towns. By 3000 BC there was the growth of "true" cities. After that, for almost 2,000 years, there was no growth of cities. It was only during the Greco-Roman times that cities came into existence. New cities appeared in new regions and the old ones disappeared. The cities of Mesopotamia, India and Egypt, Persia, Greece and Rome, fell because they were agricultural. The cities of Western Europe went on increasing. Since 1800, the rate of growth of urbanization went on at a fast pace. The 19th century was a period of true urban revolution.

Urbanization is the growth of cities and towns. It is a process of becoming urban-moving to cities, changing from agricultural to other nonagricultural occupations and thereby basic changes in the thinking and behavior patterns and social values of the people. Today, increasing number of people are living in urban areas.

The growth of cities may be due to various factors. They are classified on the basis of their major activity. For example, they could be classified as defense cities, commercial cities, production centers or manufacturing or industrial cities, political cities, religious cities, educational cities, resort cities and so on. But, today's city performs a number of activities though a particular city may have grown due to one factor initially. Some of the factors responsible for the growth of cities are surplus resources, industrialization and commercialization, development of transport and communication, economic pull and employment opportunities of the city and educational and recreational facilities.

## ■ FEATURES OF URBAN COMMUNITY

1. *Social Heterogeneity*—The city has a variety of people and groups, each representing a different culture. There is a variety of personal traits, occupations and ideas of the urban community. According to Louis Wirth "the city has been the melting pot of races, peoples and cultures and a most favorable breeding ground of new biological and cultural hybrids." The city is a complex community with different ways of thinking, behaving, acting, habits, morals, religious practices and beliefs, food and dress habits, occupations, etc., among its people.
2. *Large Size, High Density of Population, Secondary Relations and Namelessness (anonymity)*—The city is large in size i.e. spread over a large area and having a large population, which means density of population is high. Therefore, the city cannot have primary relations. They do not have the sense of belongingness to any group. The city is a secondary group, with secondary relations. The people do not have very close or intimate relations with each other. The city dwellers treat the strangers as animated machines rather than as human beings. A person may be living in a city for several years but may not know the names of the people, who live in the neighborhood. They have impersonal relations, a lack of community feeling and maintain a social distance.
3. *Homelessness*—Housing is a major problem in the city. The city is characterized by a large population, with a high density of

population. This leads to problems of housing and the growth of slums.
4. *Class Extremes*—The city is a case of extremes, with the very rich and very poor living together. The best forms of ethical behavior and the worst racketeering, superior creativeness and chronic unemployment, etc., are found existing together in the urban areas.
5. *Social Mobility*—There is a large scale mobility in urban areas. Social mobility refers to the movement of people from one social status to another. The social status of an individual is determined by his achievements and not by heredity. There are no restrictions on the individual's life. Therefore, urban life becomes more competitive and stressful. This makes the people more individualistic.
6. *Secondary Controls*—The traditional informal social controls like customs, traditions, religion, etc., loose their importance for the individual. They are no longer able to control the behavior of the individuals. Therefore, stronger formal social controls like law, police, courts, etc., are required to control the behavior of the individuals.
7. *Individuality*-The individuals develop a personality of their own. They are more individualistic, egoistic and selfish because of the growth of voluntary associations and secondary controls in the city.
8. *Voluntary Associations*—The people in the city are not traditional and orthodox. Therefore, new associations are formed, as they are more individualistic, rational, educated and conscious about their rights.
9. *Lack of Unity in the Family and Moral Laxity*—There is a great individuality in the urban family. The members do not interfere in others lives. Moral laxity is greater because of the lack of traditional social controls, western influence, the nuclear family, etc.
10. *Unbalanced Personality*—The urban personality is unbalanced due to the combination of untrue facts, looseness in character, morals, artificial environment, the influence of movies and other forms of entertainment and the atmosphere of luxury and comfort.

11. *Social Disorganization and Higher Incidence of Crime*—There are greater conflicts in urban areas, which effect the mental and physical health of the people, leading to social disorganization. This results in a higher incidence of crime in the cities.
12. *Dynamic Life*—Greater and faster changes are observed in all aspects of urban life. Therefore, urban life is more dynamic.
13. *Division of Labor and Specialization*—There is a greater specialization in all aspects of life. Thus, there is greater division and sharing of work, delegation of authority and segmentation of responsibility.

## CITY COMMUNITY IN INDIA

The city community in India has existed from ancient times. Ancient Indian history mentions a number of cities like Ayodhya, Magadha, Pataliputra, Taxila, Ujjain and others. The word "Pura" was used originally to mean a "fortified place". Later or it came to be used as a suffix to denote "a city" like Nagpur, Solapur, Manipur, etc. The number of cities were few in the ancient times. The growth of cities in India resulted from large-scale immigration from the villages and the spread of industrialization. The increase in urban population has resulted in the increase in urban areas. Compared to England and United States, the urban population in India is very small. Some of the most populated cities in India are Mumbai, Delhi, Kolkatta, Chennai and Bangalore.

## URBAN-RURAL CONTRAST

Urbanization is the growth of cities and towns. It is a process of becoming urban. Today, increasing number of people are living in urban areas. Industrialization and modernization are accompanied by the growth of cities. The village is also affected by the growth and expansion of the city. Inspite of the influence of urbanization, the villages still have their traditional features. Thus, there is a sharp contrast between the urban and rural communities. Some of the distinguishing features of the urban and rural communities are the following:

| Features | Urban community | Rural community |
|---|---|---|
| Size | Large in size, with a high density of population. | Small in size, with the number of people living in it being very few i.e. low density of population. |
| Population | Heterogeneous community with a variety of people living together. There are more social differences. | Homogenous community, with unity and uniformity in their social life. Less social differential stratification. |
| Occupation | Nonagricultural occupations and greatly interdependent in organization. | Agriculture and some small scale activities and crafts. They are generally self-sufficient units. |
| Environment | Live in artificially created atmosphere, with a lot of tensions and strains. | Live in a natural environment. They are close to nature, free from mental tensions and strains. |
| Social relations, Social contacts and Social distance | Secondary impersonal relationships. Lack of community feeling and maintain social distance. Live like strangers and anonymity develops. | Primary, personal, informal and intimate relationships. Strong community feeling or "we" feeling. Neighborhood feeling is greater. |
| Social and Physical mobility | There is a large scale social as, well as physical mobility. | Social mobility is low due to certain social conditions and restrictions. Physical mobility is low due to lack of transport and communication. |
| Family | Family is less stable and more modern. The small family is the norm. Nuclear family consists of the parents and unmarried children only. | Joint family is a very important and dominant institution. More stable family. Family is large consisting of all blood relations. |
| Marriage | More freedom in the selection of mates. Divorce is more common. | Arranged marriage by elders is more common. Divorce is rare. |

*Contd...*

*Contd...*

| Features | Urban community | Rural community |
|---|---|---|
| Status of Women | Equal status and opportunities with the men. More educated, independent and carrier conscious. | Low status, ignorant, suppressed and lack of freedom. |
| Educational Levels | Formal, advanced and widespread education. | Less formal and less importance to education. |
| Economic Status | A number of classes come into existence and class conflicts increase. | Not much of class differences and therefore, less class consciousness and class conflicts. |
| Religion | Religion becomes less important. | Rigid religious beliefs. |
| Culture | Variety of cultures, secular and cosmopolitan. | Conservative and ethnocentric. |
| Recreational Activities | Variety of recreational activities. | Simple and limited essential activities. |
| Social Controls | Formal means of social controls like law, courts, police, etc., required to control the behavior of people. | Informal means of social controls like religion, customs, traditions, etc., are enough to control the behavior of the people. |

## ■ MAJOR URBAN PROBLEMS

*The growth of cities and towns*—Urbanization is taking place at a very fast pace. Some of the factors responsible for this growth are the processes of industrialization, migration, economic factors, political factors, religious and educational factors, transport and communication facilities, cultural centers, means of entertainment, art centers, business centers, etc., in under-developed countries like India. The rapid rate of growth of cities has resulted in unplanned urbanization, giving rise to a number of problems. Some of the major urban problems are the following:

1. *Concentration of Population*—There is a heavy concentration of population in urban areas. The density of population is very high in the cities.

2. *Problem of Slums and Unplanned Growth of Cities*—One of the consequences of overcrowding is the growth of slums in the cities. A slum is a building, group of buildings or area characterized by overcrowding, with deterioration in civic amenities, unsanitary and unhygienic conditions of living, where the poverty stricken people, ill fed and ill clad children, the diseased, the addicts, beggars, criminals and prostitutes live. This is one of the major problems of urbanization.
3. *Lack of Facilities*—Besides the problem of slums and overcrowding, there are lack of basic facilities of housing, water and fresh air, improper sanitation, leading to poor drainage and hygienic conditions. Along with this, there is also an acute power shortage.
4. *Transport and Traffic*—With the increase in population and overcrowding, there is an increase in both private and public vehicles, which increases the traffic and noise pollution in the urban areas. Also, there are no sufficient transport facilities for the growing population.
5. *Problem of Privacy*—There is a lack of privacy and intimacy in the city due to the secondary relations. People are impersonal and indifferent towards each other. They become more selfish, individualistic and calculative.
6. *Family Disorganization*—The traditional joint family is disintegrating, giving way to modern nuclear family. The small family norm is now observed in the city. Divorce, desertion and separation are increasing.
7. *Social Controls and Social Deviance*—The traditional social controls of religion, beliefs, customs and traditions, joint family, caste, etc., are loosing their importance for the city dwellers. Thus, social deviance is increasing. The city life has become uncertain, insecure and competitive.
8. *Problem of Vices*—The city is said to be the center of economic insecurity, mental illness, gambling, prostitution, drunkenness, crime, juvenile delinquency, alcoholism, environmental pollution, etc., coupled with poverty.
9. *Health Problems*—Some of the common diseases in urban areas are respiratory diseases, fever, gastrointestinal tract (GIT) disorders, skin infection, eye infections, viral infections, chronic toxicity, sexually transmilited diseases (STD), etc., which are caused due to

industrial pollution, over crowding, poor hygienic conditions and practices, food and water contamination, poverty, unemployment and malnutrition. In order to improve the health of the city dweller, the basic necessities have to be provided like safe drinking water, maintaining housing standards, proper disposal of liquid and solid waste and conducting health awareness campaigns.

## ■ THE REGIONAL COMMUNITY

A region is an important social unit. The term "region" means a geographical area, where the society is held together for a length of time, with common cultural and linguistic characteristics. The people of each region therefore have their own way of life and resemble each other. Lundberge defines a region as "an area within which the people and the different constituent communities are conspicuously more inter-dependent than they are with the people of other areas." The boundaries of a region may or may not be the same as that of the state or the nation. It usually combines rural and urban communities into one and exhibits the characteristics of both the rural and the urban community. A region must be a balanced and integrated community.

India has a number of regions, which have a geographic cultural and linguistic significance. Regionalism is the community feeling within a region. It gives man a feeling of oneness with the fellow human beings. It implies an integral relationship with a larger whole, as will as involves a cultural wholeness.

Regionalism has some advantages and disadvantages also. Sometimes, it may affect the national unity and integration. People of the same region will help each other and work for their own group welfare. It promotes regional development and cultural growth. Regionalism effects the economic progress of the nation and effects the national development.

### Regions in India

India is broadly divided into the following regions — southern region, western region, northern region and eastern region. Southern region includes Karnataka, Tamil Nadu, Andhra Pradesh and Kerala. Western region includes Maharashtra and Gujarat. Northern region includes

Jammu and Kashmir, Punjab, Rajasthan, Uttar Pradesh and Delhi. Eastern region includes Assam, Orrissa, Bihar and West Bengal.

These regions have been created to discuss economic and other matters of mutual interests. Each state within the regions has its own language, culture and social problems, which become a barrier in the development of the regions. For example, the feud between Karnataka and Tamil Nadu over the sharing of Cauvery water, proves the absence of community feeling among the states in the same region.

### POINTS TO NOTE
1. Meaning and features of urban community
2. City or urban India
3. Urban rural contrast
4. Major urban and health problems
5. Regional community—Division of the country in to different Zones- East- West-North-South.

### NURSING IMPLICATIONS
The study of the urban community will help the nurse to understand the environment or living conditions of the individual. Health consequences and problems of the urban atmosphere and the social problems. The effect of the regional differences on the social and cultural life of the people.

### QUESTIONS
1. Problems of the rural community.
2. Health problems of rural community.
3. Discuss the rural-urban contrast.
4. Health problem of urban community.
5. Urban social problems.
6. Features of Indian villages.
7. Describe the characteristics of the rural community.
8. Discuss the urban social and health problems.
9. What are the social consequences of urbanization in India?
10. Explain the causes of the growth of urbanization in India.
11. Write a short note on regional community.

# 9. Social Stratification

- Class and caste
- The Indian caste system
- Origin of caste
- Outstanding features
- Caste in India today
- Features of caste system in India
- Social mobility

## ■ CLASS AND CASTE

Social stratification and social differentiation are two most important social processes found in most of the societies. Differentiation is there in all human societies. This gives rise to diversity and irregularities in the society. Thus, human society is stratified everywhere.

Social stratification is the social arrangement of groups of people in the society in a higher and lower status and who enjoy privileges and suffer disabilities according to their status. Social stratification will be there in the society as long as social irregularities persist and so long as they are consequential for the life-chances and lifestyle of different strata that make up any society. The members of any society are arranged in terms of superiority, inferiority and equality. This arrangement of people in strata or layers is called as social stratification.

### Definition

1. P Gisbert defines social stratification as "the division of the society into permanent groups of categories linked with each other by the relationship of superiority and subordination".
2. According to Raymond W Murray social stratification is "a horizontal division of society into higher and lower social units."
3. According to Ogburn and Nimkoff social stratification is "a process by which individuals and groups are ranked in a more or less enduring hierarchy of status."

4. Melvin M Tumin refers to social stratification as "an arrangement of any social group or society into a hierarchy of positions that are unequal with regard to power, property, social evaluation or psychic gratification."

From the above definition given by Melvin M Tumin, the characteristics of social stratification are as follows:
1. It is social i.e. patterned in character. It is not a biological inequality.
2. It is ancient i.e. it has been found in all societies at all times from the ancient times.
3. It is ubiquitous, i.e. it is a universal and a worldwide phenomenon.
4. It is diverse in its forms. It is based on different factors. For example, caste, class and esteem are the most common forms of stratification in the modern world.
5. It is consequential i.e. the most important, most desired and often scarcest things in human life are distributed unequally. This leads to two main kinds of consequences - life chances and life styles.

There are certain factors that determine social stratification in any society like the basic differences among human beings, necessity of different functions and need for a social equilibrium. The basis for social stratification may be categorized as biological and sociocultural. The biological bases depend on biological distinctions like sex, age, race and birth. The sociocultural bases for social stratification are economic status, political power and religious power. On the basis of above mentioned biological and sociocultural factors, the general forms of social stratification are caste stratification, class stratification and race stratification.

## ■ THE INDIAN CASTE SYSTEM

The caste system, the joint family system and the village system are considered to be the three basic pillars of the Indian social system. The caste system is a peculiar feature of the Hindu society in India. The word "caste" owes its origin to the Spanish word "casta" meaning "breed, race, strain or a complex of hereditary qualities". The Portuguese applied this term to the classes of people in India known by the name "jati". The Sanskrit word for the caste is "varna" meaning "color". The caste system owes its origin to the Varna system of the Hindu society, which is based on the division of labor and occupation. The caste system is supposed to have had a divine origin and sanction. There are at least about 3,000 castes and sub-castes in India.

## Definition

Caste is a peculiar and complex phenomenon, which is difficult to define. Different writers have defined it in different ways by taking its characteristics into consideration.
1. Herbert Risley has defined caste as "a collection of families, bearing a common name, claiming a common descent, from a mythical ancestor, human or divine, professing to follow the same hereditary calling, and regarded by those who are competent to give an opinion, as forming a single homogenous community."
2. CH Cooley says "when a class is somewhat hereditary, we may call it a caste."
3. According to Mac Iver and Page, "when status is wholly predetermined so that men are born to their lot, without any hope of changing it, then class takes the extreme form of caste."
4. SC Dube says that "caste is an endogamous unity with more or less defined rituals, status and some occupation traditionally linked to it."
5. Henry Maine forms an opinion that "castes started as natural division of occupational classes and eventually upon receiving the religious sanction, became solidified into the existing caste system. The caste system comes into being when it becomes an integral part of a religious dogma, which divides the people into superior and inferior groups, with different responsibilities, functions and standards of living."
6. Ketker says "a caste is a group having two characteristics (i) membership is confined to those who are born of members and includes all persons so born. (ii) members are forbidden by an inexorable social law to marry outside the group."
7. DM Majumdar and TN Madan have described caste as "a closed group".
8. According to Green, "caste is a system of stratification in which mobility, up and down the status ladder, at least ideally may not occur."

9. According to Megasthenes, the Greek traveler, who visited India in the third century BC, observed two important elements of the caste system in India (i) there is no inter marriage, and (ii) there can be no change of profession.

## Features or Characteristics of the Caste System

Dr GS Ghurye has made a detailed study of the caste system in India. He has come to the conclusion that there is no real general definition of caste because of its complex nature. Therefore, according to him the best way to understand the term "caste" is to study the various factors underlying the caste system. To get a complete idea of what caste is, the traditional features of the caste system as described by Dr Ghurye are the following:

1. *Hierarchical Division of the Society*—The Hindu society is divided into small groups and sub groups called the castes and sub castes. These groups have a hierarchical position in the society, with the Brahmin at the top of the hierarchy and the Shudra at the bottom of the hierarchy. The Kshatriya and the Vaishya have an intermediary position in the social scale. An individual born into a particular caste cannot change his caste status till his death. He remains in his caste status throughout his life.
2. *Segmental Division of the Society*—The Hindu society is divided into a number of segments called "castes". The membership into these castes is dependent on birth. The status of the individual is dependent upon the traditional importance of the caste into which he had the fortune of being born. Thus, caste is hereditary and therefore, nothing can change his caste status. Each caste has its own way of life, with its own custom traditions, practices and rituals. It has its own informal rules, regulations and procedures. There were the "cast councils" or "caste panchayats" to control and regulate the conduct of caste members.
3. *Caste Panchayat*—Every caste has its own caste panchayat. It is the governing body of the caste, which literally means a body of five members but in fact there are many more who meet whenever decisions have to be taken. It used to perform a number of functions. It regulates and controls the conduct of all caste members. Caste Panchayat is a very powerful organization and rules over the whole caste. The panchayat would also settle disputes

and give its final verdict on the issues referred to it. It would decide civil and criminal matters and would give punishment to those who violated caste rules and obligations. Its chief punishments were in the form of fines, feast to be given to caste men, corporal punishment, religious expiation like taking bath in holy waters and out casting. In short "caste is its own ruler". The caste panchayat was also striving to promote the welfare of the caste members and safe guarding the interests of the caste members.

4. *Restrictions on Feeding*—The caste system lays down a number of restrictions on the food habits of the members in order to preserve the ceremonial purity of the superior castes. For example, who should accept what kind of food and from whom - is often decided by the caste. A Brahmin will accept "pakka" food only i.e. food cooked in ghee from any caste, but he will accept "kaccha" food i.e. food cooked with water, only from his own caste people. Generally, as a matter of rule and practice, no individual belonging to a higher caste will accept "kaccha" food prepared by an individual belonging to a lower caste.

5. *Restrictions on Social Relations*—The caste system puts restrictions on the extent of social relations. Thus, there are restrictions with regard to distances that the people of the lower caste had to maintain with the higher caste. This gave rise to the theory of pollution communicated by some castes to the members of the higher castes. For example, in Kerala, a Nair may approach a Namboodri Brahmin, but must not touch him, while Tiyan must keep himself at a distance of 36 steps from the Brahmin and Pulayan at a distance of 96 steps. This has resulted in the practice of untouchability in the Indian society. It has also lead to the segregation of the lower caste people from the rest of the society.

6. *Social and Religious Disabilities of Certain Castes*—The theory of pollution and the consequent practice of untouchability in the traditional caste society, resulted in the lower caste people like the shudras, suffering from a number of social and religious disabilities. They could not use the public roads, draw water from the public wells, enter the Hindu temples, attend public schools and were generally made to live on the outskirts of the city or the village.

7. *Civil and Religious Privileges of Certain Castes*—The upper castes like the Brahmins, Kshatriyas and Vaishyas enjoyed certain civil

and religious privileges in the society because of their caste status. They have more freedom because they are supposed to be more superior. Education and teaching, chanting of Vedic Mantras and other religious texts were the privileges of the Brahmin caste only. The upper castes in general enjoyed all social, political, religious and legal privileges.

8. *Restrictions on the Choice of Occupation*—There are restrictions on the choice of occupation of the individual. Every caste had its occupation and the individual had to take up the occupation of the caste into which he was born. Occupations were almost hereditary and they could not change to other occupations of their liking. Some occupations like learning, priesthood, teaching, which the Brahmins pursued, were considered to be prestigious and sacred occupations while certain other occupations like that of barbers, washer men, shoemaking, tanning and curing of hides, sweeping, etc., were considered to be the dirty and degrading jobs of the society, which was done by the lower castes like the shudras.

9. *Restrictions on Marriage*—The caste system lays down restrictions on marriage also. Caste is an endogamous group. In fact, sociologists regard endogamy as the very essence of the caste system. Endogamy is a rule of marriage according to which an individual has to marry within his own caste. Each caste is subdivided into subgroups called as subcastes and each of these subcastes are also endogamous. For example, Iyers, Iyengars, Madhvas, Smarthas, etc., are all Brahmin subcastes, which are endogamous. According to this rule therefore, intercaste marriages are forbidden. But, the caste provides for some kind of exogamous marriages.

*Exogamy*—Exogamy is the opposite of endogamy. Exogamy is a rule of marriage according to which an individual has to marry outside one's own group. Marriage is prohibited within one's own group. Sapinda, Sagothra and Sapravara marriages have been generally forbidden by the upper castes in the Hindu society.

1. *Sapinda Exogamy*—Among Hindus, marriage within the Pinda is prohibited. There are different opinions about who can be said to be belonging to same Pinda. According to the Mitakshara School, those who are the descendents of a common parentage are said to be belonging to the same Pinda. According to Bruhaspati,

offsprings from five maternal generations and seven paternal generations are said to be Spinda and they cannot intermarry. Generally, Sapinda marriages do not take place and Sapinda exogamy is followed in India.

2. *Sagotra Exogamy*—Sagotra Exogamy is followed by most of the upper castes like Brahmins and Kshatriyas of the caste society. Sagotra exogamy is the marriage outside one's own gotra and marriage within the gotra is prohibited. This restriction is followed because people of the same gotra are believed to have similar blood.

3. *Sapravara Exogamy*—Pravaras are the name of saints. Sapravara marriages are forbidden especially among the Brahmins. People who utter the name of a common saint at religious functions are believed to be belonging to the same pravara. Therefore, persons belonging to same pravara cannot intermarry. Thus, pravara is a religious and spiritual bond. Sapravara exogamy i.e. marriage outside one's own pravara has been imposed as a rule for the upper caste, especially the Brahmins.

## ORIGIN OF CASTE SYSTEM

Caste system is a peculiar and a complex phenomenon existing in India since ancient times. A number of theories have been put forward by social thinkers to explain its origin. Some of the most important theories are the traditional theory, occupational theory, religious theory, political theory, racial theory and evolutionary theory.

Caste system is supposed to have originated from the chaturvarna system, according to which the Hindu society was divided into four main Varnas namely the Brahmins, the Kshatriyas, the Vaishyas and the Shudras. The Varna system was prevalent during the Vedic Period. It was based on the principle of division of labor and occupations. Varnas and castes are not the same. According to Prof G S Ghurye "caste in India must be regarded as a Brahminic child of the Indo-Aryan culture, cradled in the land of Ganges and then transferred to the other parts of India by the Brahmin prospectors." Classes mentioned in the Rig Veda are based on the division of labor i.e. occupations adopted by the groups. Therefore, they were not stratified or rigid.

During the post-Vedic and Medieval Period, caste developed into a rigid and stratified institution based on birth, imposing a number of restrictions on the relations between them. During the Modern period, several changes have taken place in the structure and functions of caste. Some of the factors that have facilitated the existence and the growth of caste system in India are the geographic isolation, static society, rural social structure, aggregation of people, influence of religions, difference of races, lack of education, existence of many races, clashes between them, hereditary occupations, desire of the Brahmins to keep themselves pure, ideas of exclusive family, ancestor worship, sacramental meal deliberate economic and administrative policies followed by various conquerors, especially the British, color prejudices and conquest, etc.

# CASTE IN INDIA TODAY

## Merits and Demerits of Caste System

The Indian caste system has its own merits and demerits.

## Merits of Caste System

1. Caste is based on the division of labor and occupation. Therefore, there is harmony in the society.
2. Spirit of cooperation and fellow feeling develops among the people of the same caste, which strengthens the group sentiment. This is helpful for the poor and the needy.
3. Caste is a source of social stability. Social stability of the Indian society is maintained by caste.
4. Caste acts as a constitution of the Hindu society.
5. Racial purity is maintained by castes due to its endogamous nature.
6. Caste provides for the transmission of culture. Caste culture is passed on from one generation to the next generation.
7. Caste decides the career and provides for the profession of the individual.

Thus, caste takes care of all the individual's necessities, from the time of his birth till his death.

## Demerits of the Caste System

1. Caste has given rise to the evil system of untouchability in the Indian society due to the concept of purity and pollution practiced in the caste system.
2. Caste system has divided the Hindu society, retarding the growth of solidarity and brotherhood and denying any type of social intercourse between them.
3. It has hindered the growth of the spirit of national consciousness and national unity and the proper growth of democracy.
4. Political disunity is created due to caste feelings.
5. Caste has retarded progress.
6. There is restriction of social mobility.
7. It has lowered the status of women.
8. It has given scope for conversion especially of the lower castes to the other religions due to the oppression and suppression by the upper castes.
9. *Casteism*—Casteism has increased in the society due to very strong feelings of caste. Casteism is a blind group loyalty towards one's own caste or sub-caste, which does not care for the interests of other castes and seeks to realize the social, economic, political and other interests of its own group. Casteism ignores the healthy social standards of justice, fair play, equity and brotherhood. Under the influence of casteism, members of one caste do not hesitate to harm the interests of the members of the other castes. Casteism has led to caste clashes and lot of destruction in the society.
10. *Health*—The health of the under-privileged sections of the caste system gets effected due to their lower status in the caste society. This is due to poverty, social stigma, overcrowding, illiteracy, beliefs, traditions, cultural barriers, unhygienic conditions of living in slums, with poor sanitation, low standards of living, etc. All these conditions lead to occurrence of communicable diseases and epidemics.

## ■ FEATURES OF CASTE SYSTEM IN INDIA

### Interdependence of Castes (Jajmani System)

Caste system, as discussed above, in its traditional form, is a peculiar feature of the Hindu society in India. It has a number of rules of social behavior, which cannot be violated and which maintains control over its members. Although the different castes are socially segregated, on several occasions, one caste has to secure the services of the other castes. Such dependency among the castes has been called as "vertical unity" by Prof MN Srinivas.

It has also been given the name of "jajmani system" under which each group of the village is expected to give certain standardized services to the other castes. It is a functional interdependence of castes. The system is based on economic interests and fulfillment of needs and requirements of the caste groups. For example, Brahmins will perform various religious services for the other castes or the barber or the dhobi or the kumhar or the darji or the chamar rendering their services for the upper caste groups. Thus, the jajmani system is based on the barter system. Most of these relations are permanent and hereditary. In its traditional form, it provided economic security and security of occupation. But, in modern India, it has been reduced to an exploitation of the lower castes by the upper castes. Due to the impact of industrialization, urbanization and the development of the means of transport and communication, this system is disintegrating.

## Changing Trends in the Caste System

Caste system is described as a rigid system. But, inspite of its rigid rules and regulations for the behavior of its members, a number of changes can be observed in the caste system. This is because society is never static. Conditions in the society are constantly changing and the social system must adjust to the changing conditions. Some of the most important factors responsible for bringing about changes in the caste system are the impact of modern education introduced by the British, the reformist movements, legislation during the British rule, industrialization, urbanization, westernization, technological advancement, improved transport and communication system, improvement in the status of women, evolution of new social classes, division of labor, etc.

## Social Class

Class is an universal phenomenon found in almost all modern societies. According to Ogburn and Nimkoff "a social class is the aggregate of persons having essentially the same social status in a given society." It is based on economic considerations and other personal and individual attainments. Members of a particular class have a status attached to them and the corresponding roles to play. Accordingly, relations of superiority and inferiority develop among the classes. In such a society, there is greater social mobility i.e. there is a possibility of the people moving up or down the social scale in the society. Classes may be determined on the criterion of birth or wealth or occupation or polity or education.

## Class and Caste–Differences

| Class | Caste |
| --- | --- |
| Membership is based on various factors like wealth, education, occupation, etc. | Membership is based on birth. |
| Status is achieved | Status is ascribed |
| Social stratification is an open system, i.e. members can change their class. | Social stratification is closed, i.e. members cannot change their caste. |
| Flexible system of stratification. | Rigid system of stratification. |
| Not sacred, more secular in origin. It does not hinder democracy. | Believed to have been divinely ordained. It is religious and sacred. It hinders democracy. |
| Greater freedom and no restrictions for the members, i.e. exogamous. | Endogamous i.e. marriage and social relationships have to be within one's own caste. |
| Feeling of class consciousness is necessary to constitute a class. | No need for any subjective consciousness among the members. |
| No rigidly fixed order of prestige of the classes. | Prestige of the different castes is well established. |
| Feeling of disparity among the members. | Idea of purity and impurity among the members giving rise to the concept of untouchability. |
| Less social distance among the members and greater tolerance for each other. | Social distance is maintained among the members. |
| More progressive. | Conservative. |
| Greater social mobility. | Less social mobility. |

## ■ SOCIAL MOBILITY

Social stratification and social differentiation are two most important social processes found in most societies. Individuals and classes are accordingly ranked high or low in the social scale of the society on the basis of the characteristics possessed by them according to the social value scale. Any change in the value scale or any change in the characteristics results in a change in the status of the individuals and the classes.

Social change is universal. The society and the individuals are dynamic. Individual would always be striving to enhance their status in the society by moving from a lower position to a higher position. Many times, people of higher status also may be forced to come down to a lower status. Thus, it is seen that people in the society continue to move up and down the status scale. This movement of people is called social mobility.

Social mobility is the movement of people or groups of people from one social status or position to another status or position. For example, a poor person may become rich or a shopkeeper may become a minister, a small business man may become an industrialist and so on. On the other hand, it may also happen that the businessman becomes a bankrupt or the minister loses his job and comes back to his old shop and so on.

### Kinds of Social Mobility

Social mobility is of two types
  i. Vertical Social mobility.
  ii. Horizontal Social Mobility.

  i. *Vertical Mobility*—Vertical mobility refers to the movement of people from one status to another, which may involve a change in class, occupation or power. This movement may be upward or downward on the status scale. For example, the upward movement of the poor class to the middle class or the downward movement of a minister who loses his job and comes back to his original job of a shopkeeper.
  ii. *Horizontal Mobility*—Horizontal mobility refers to a change in the position without any change in the status like a change in the residence or job without any change in the status. For example,

a teacher leaving one school to work in another school or an engineer taking up a job in another factory.

### POINTS TO NOTE
1. The Indian caste system-definition-origin-features.
2. Merits and demerits of caste system.
3. Jajmani systems.
4. Class system–features–changes from caste to class system in India.
5. Adverse effects of caste-social mobility in India.

### NURSING IMPLICATIONS
Knowledge about the caste system gives an in-depth knowledge of the life of the people of India. It controls the individual life from birth to death especially among the Hindus who form a major portion of the population. It has an impact on the social economic political and cultural life of the people.

### QUESTIONS
1. Define:
    a. Caste and class
    b. Casteism
    c. Varna system
    d. Jajmani System
    e. Social mobility
    f. Social distance and social mobility
2. Social distance and social mobility.
3. Changes in the caste system.
4. Origin of caste.
5. Adverse effects of caste.
6. Describe social stratification and show its peculiar nature in India.
7. Define social stratification. What is the basis of social stratification?
8. Define class and caste. Discuss the caste system in India.
9. Explain the features of the traditional Indian caste system.
10. Explain the changes that have taken place in the caste system.
11. Differentiate between class and caste.
12. List out the adverse effects of the caste. What are its consequences on health?

# CHAPTER 10

# Social System

- Definition of a social system
- Principle types of social systems
- Role and status

## ■ MEANING

Social system is related to the concept of social structure. Social structure is one of the basic concepts of Sociology. Man being a social animal, cannot live alone. He interacts with other human beings. These interactions result in the formation of groups, organizations, associations, institutions and communities. These are the structural forms of the society. They are arranged in an interrelated way to enable the society to function in a harmonious manner. The functions of the society are carried out through these structural units.

A social system is an orderly and systematic arrangement of social interactions. The individuals are a part of the social system. They interact with each other, influencing each others behavior patterns. Their behavior is controlled by the norms of the society. The groups thus formed are a part of the larger society. They do not act in an isolated and independent manner. A social system is thus formed on the basis of these interactions and interrelationships.

"System" refers to an orderly arrangement of parts. Social system refers to an orderly arrangement of the components of the society viz human interactions. Individuals influence each other during these interactions. These inter-actions and inter-relationships assume a definite pattern which is a social system. It also refers to the analysis of groups, institutions, societies and intersocietal entities. For example, a university or the state may be referred to as a system.

The parts of the social system are related to each other on the basis of the functional aspect. Social system relates to the functional aspect of the social structure. Social structure is the means through which the social system functions.

## Definition

1. According to Talcott Parsons, a social system "consists in a plurality of individual actors, interacting with each other in a situation, which has at least a physical or environmental aspect, actors who are motivated in terms of a tendency to the optimization of gratification and whose relation to this situations, including each other, is defined and mediated in terms of a system of culturally structured and shared symbols."
2. WF Ogburn defines it as "a plurality of individuals interacting with each other according to shared cultural norms and meaning."
3. According to David Popenoe, "a social system is a set of persons or groups, who interact with one another; the set is conceived of as a social unit distinct from the particular persons who compose it."
4. In his "A dictionary of Sociology", Duncan Mitchell writes "a social system basically consists of two or more individuals, interacting directly or indirectly, in a bounded situation."

Thus, the term "Social System" in Sociology has been evolved to study the society. According to Max Weber, it represents an "ideal type".

## Characteristics of Social System

From the above definitions, the main characteristics of a social system are the following:
1. *Social System is Based on Social Interaction*—Social system requires at least two or more individuals interacting with each other. A single individual alone cannot make up a social system. The interactions between a number of individuals produce a system which is called a "social system".
2. *The Interaction Should be Meaningful* —The human interactions create social relationships, which find their expression in traditions, customs, mores, laws, institutions, etc. Social system is an organization of these various expressions of social relationships. Aimless and meaningless interactions do not produce a social system.
3. *Social System is a Unity*—Social system is a state or condition where the various expressions of social relationships are arranged in an integrated manner. It implies an order among the interacting

units of the system. Any arrangement of the above expressions does not constitute a social system.
4. *Parts of the Social System are Related on the Basis of the Functional Relationship*—The different parts of the social system are united to each other on the basis of the functional relationship. Each part has its assigned role and performs its function. It is an arrangement of interdependent and interactive parts based on the functional relationship.
5. *Social System is Related to the Cultural System*—Cultural system consists of the norms and values of the individuals in the system. This culture determines the nature and scope of the interrelations and interactions of the individuals in the system. It maintains a balance and harmonious relationship among the different parts of the system. Thus, the social system is closely related to the cultural system.
6. *Social System has an Environmental Aspect and the Quality of Self-adjustments*—Social system is dynamic and it is not static. It is not the same at all times, territories and societies. Social system changes with change in time. It does not disturb the social equilibrium. Inspite of the social changes, the social system continues to exist and has the quality of self-adjustment. For example, changes in the family system getting adjusted to changes in the society.

## ■ PRINCIPAL TYPES OF SOCIAL SYSTEM

Some of the principal types of social systems have been studied by social thinkers like Morgan, Dukheim, Sorokin and others
1. *Classification by Morgan and other Evolutionists*—Evolutionists have classified the social systems on the basis of evolution. According to them, society or social system has passed through these stages
   i. Savagery
   ii. Barbarian
   iii. Civilized Social Systems
   They have also classified social systems on the basis of the means of livelihood as
   a. Hunting
   b. Pastoral

c. Agricultural
   d. Industrial social systems
2. *Durkheim's Classification*—According to Durkheim, there are two types of social systems:
   i. Mechanical social system of the ancient times.
   ii. Organic social system found in the modern societies.
3. *Sorokin's Classification*—Sorokin classifies the social system on the basis of culture. According to him, there are three types of cultural systems, which are:
   i. Sensate cultural system where material happiness is given importance.
   ii. Ideational cultural system, where spiritual happiness is given importance.
   iii. Idealistic cultural system, where both material and spiritual happiness are given importance.

## Elements of the Social System

The concept of social system is closely related to the concept of social structure. Social system is the functional aspect of the social structure. Social structure is the means through which the social system functions. A social system is formed on the basis of the interactions and interrelationships of the individuals. Thus, the individual is the basic element in the social system. The social system is formed by the actions of the individuals. The individuals have to participate in the process of interaction. This involves two important aspects - the positional aspect and the processional aspect.

The Positional aspect is the position of the individual, i.e. the actor in the social system, which is his status. The processional aspect is the functional importance of the actor or individual in the social system, which is called the role that the individual has to play in the social system in accordance with his status in the social system. Thus, there are three elements of the social system - the social act or action, the actor and the status-role.

*The Social Act or Action*—The social act or action is a process in the social system, which motivates the individual or individuals in the case of a group. The orientation of the action has a bearing on the attainment of gratifications or the avoidance of deprivations of the actor. The actor has certain needs and thus develops a system of expectations according to his needs. The needs of the individual actor have two aspects - the gratificational aspect and the orientational aspect. The gratification aspect is concerned with what the actor gets out of his interaction and what its costs are to him. The orientational aspect is concerned with "how" he gets it. Both these aspects must be present in what is called a "social act" or "action".

*The Actors*—The actor is an important element of the social system. He has a certain status and the corresponding role to perform in the system. The social system must have a sufficient proportion of its component actors adequately motivated to act in accordance with the requirements of its role system. The social system also must be adapted to the minimum needs of the individual actors. The system must secure sufficient participation of its actors also. In other words, it must motivate them adequately to the performances, which are necessary for the social system to develop or persist. The actor has to act according to the roles assigned to him. This he learns through the process of socialization. Through the process of social control, the social system limits and regulates the needs and actions of the actor. The act and the actor are thus complementary to each other.

*The Role and Status*—The social system consists of the interactions and interrelationships among the individuals or the actors. The participation of the actors in the process of interactive relationship has two aspects.

i. The status, i.e. the place of the actor in the social system.
ii. The role, i.e. the functional significance of the actor for the social system.

An individual may have a high or low status in the social system, and accordingly has a definite role to play. In a social system, there are different roles, which are integrated together. The actors are distributed between the various roles in the social system.

## ROLE AND STATUS

*Social Roles*—Social status and social roles are the important features of the social structure of the society. Every individual has a particular status in the society. The social role is the expected behavior of the individual in that particular status. Thus, role is the functional aspect of a status. Role and status go together. The role of an individual is dependent on his status in the society. As the status changes, the role also changes. Thus, both status and role are dynamic and constantly changing. Each status has its role to be performed. This maintains the order of the society.

## Definition

1. Elliott and Merill define roles as "the part a person plays as a result of each status."
2. According to Ogburn and Nimkoff, role is "a set of socially expected and approved behavior pattern consisting of both duties and privileges, associated with a particular position in a group."
3. A "social role" as defined by Lundberg is "a pattern of behavior expected of an individual in a certain group or situation."
4. According to K. Davis, role is "the manner in which a person actually carries out the requirements of his position."

From the above definitions, it is clear that the role is a set of behavior patterns an individual is expected to have in a certain position in the community. The order of the social system is dependent upon how efficiently and consistently each member of the different groups performs his role in the system. Roles are a series of duties i.e. they represent reciprocal relations among the individuals. Thus, a role is a pattern of attitudes, predisposing a person in a certain position to act according to the expectations of others.

*Role Conflict*—In the modern complex societies, an individual has to play different roles in different situations. These roles may be diversified and sometimes in conflict with each other. This leads to a situation where the individual is confronted by situations in which he is uncertain of his own role and that of the others. This causes disappointment and frustration, which may lead to serious personality problems. Role conflict is thus the conflict experienced by an individual at the time of role playing. For example, the role of an individual, who is doctor and the head of the family, may sometimes be in conflict with each other. He may have to sacrifice his obligations towards his family in the interest of his patients or profession.

## Social Status

Every individual in the society or the social organization has a particular status. Social status is the position of an individual within the social relationships, which makeup the society. It may be high or low. The status of an individual is considered to be high, if the role he is playing is regarded as important by the group. If the role he is playing is regarded as less important, then he will have a lower status in the society. Thus, the status of an individual is based on the perceptions and social evaluations of the others in the society. It is recognized by a pattern of symbols, actions, prestige and respect.

## Definitions

1. According to Ogburn and Nimkoff social status is "the position of an individual in the group".
2. Mac Iver and Page define status as "the social position that determines for its possessor, apart from his personal attribute or social services, a degree of respect, prestige and influence."
3. Ralph Linton says that status is "the place in a particular system, which an individual occupies at a particular time."
4. According to Robert Bierstedt, "a status is simply a position in the society or in a group."
5. HT Mazumdar states that "status is the location of the individual within the group, his place is in the social network of reciprocal obligation, privileges, duties and responsibilities."

From the above definitions, it can be stated that social status and social role are closely related. A status is the position and role is the behavior pattern connected with the status, which is socially expected and approved by the society. This is called as role performance. In this way, status and role are the two sides of the same coin.

## Types of Social Status

### Ascribed and Achieved Status

There are two ways by which the status of an individual in the society is determined. They are through the processes of ascription and achievement. There may be some societies in which status is ascribed and in some other societies it may be achieved. Most societies make use of both the ascribed and achieved status.

## Ascribed Status

Ascribed status is that position, which an individual has by virtue of his birth, without any individual effort like nationality, religion, caste, sex, age, kinship, race, etc. In such cases, the individual has a status in a particular group involuntarily and therefore, has no choice or selection. The status, which a child has at the time of his birth is his ascribed status. His potentialities at this time are least known. This ascribed status will definitely determine and limit the range of statuses, which he may subsequently achieve or try to achieve like, status of an individual in the traditional caste system of the Hindu society in India.

## Achieved Status

Achieved status is that position, which an individual has by his own efforts or capabilities or talent. The social position is acquired through his own choice like the place of an individual in an organization. The society cannot depend only on the ascribed status. All societies have some achieved statuses, though the proportion of such statuses differs from society to society and from time to time. For example, in the primitive simple societies of the past, ascribed status was given more importance but in the modem industrial, urban societies, with social changes taking place at a very fast rate, achieved status is given importance, like the occupational status.

From the above discussion, it becomes clear that social status is of great importance for the individual, as well as the society. An individual has respect by virtue of his status in the society. He may get direct or indirect advantages or disadvantages from his social status in the society. From the point of view of the society, social status constitutes the basic organization of group life. It is necessary in the specialization of functions and in the coordination of the specialized functions of a community. But it should not be rigid. It should be flexible to social changes.

## Differences between Ascribed Status and Achieved Status

| Ascribed Status | Achieved Status |
|---|---|
| By virtue of birth. | By virtue of his own efforts or talent or capabilities. |
| Status in a group is involuntary therefore no choice or selection. | Status is voluntary. It is acquired through his own choice or selections. |
| Status is given more importance in simple and primitive societies. | More importance in modern and complex societies. |

Inspite of the above difference, it can be said that both ascribed and achieved status go together in most societies. They are complementary to each other. The achieved statuses are found within the framework of the ascribed statuses.

## Relationship between Role and Status

| Status | Role |
|---|---|
| Status is determined by sociocultural factors and relative to the other members of the groups. | Role is dependent on the position and the corresponding expected behavior pattern in the community. |
| Most of the societies have a similar pattern of statuses. | Roles may take different forms in different societies. |
| Status can be understood by taking into consideration the background of the society. | Role can be understood by taking into consideration the requirements of the society. |
| Status divides the societies into different groups like ranks, etc. | No division of the society by roles. |
| Status provides prestige and respect. | Role is just the functional aspect of the status. |
| Status is only a part of the larger social system. | Role is the behavior pattern expected of the status. |

### POINTS TO NOTE
1. Social system—definition–meaning–characteristics–types and elements.
2. Role and status–definition–types of social status–ascribed and achieved status.

## NURSING IMPLICATIONS

Understanding individual roles and status in the society gives an idea of the economic status of the individual. This is very important in the treatment of the patients, which has an impact on his life and lifestyle.

## QUESTIONS

1. Define:
   a. Social system
   b. Role-conflict
   c. Life style
   d. Role and status
2. Examine the different types of social systems of the society.
3. Write a short essay on achieved status and ascribed status.

# CHAPTER 11

# Race

- Meaning and definition of race
- Determinants of race
- Types of races in India

Race is a term which has a number of meanings. Different people have given different meanings to this term. The term "race" is used synonymously with nationality. Sometimes it is also confused with language or religion or to denote the classification of human beings on the basis of skin color or it is used in a very wide sense as "human race", which includes all human beings.

But the term "race" cannot be used in the sense that is mentioned above because race is not a sociological term but a purely biological and anthropological concept. In 1950, the UNESCO replaced the term "race" with "ethnic group". Social races are composed of socially defined and significant groups. The study of social race is a fundamental aspect of the study of social structure especially of a stratified society. Thus, race is a group of intermarrying people, who are born of common ancestors, possess similar physical traits and "we" feeling. One race can be distinguished from the other on the basis of physical characteristics, which are permanent due to inbreeding. A race originates due to mutation, migration, selection and adaptation. Membership in a race is established at birth, endures for life and confers special behavioral obligations or privileges. It is not restricted by age or sex.

## ■ DEFINITIONS

1. Anthropologists define race as "a group of individuals who possess common hereditary traits, which separate them from other groups."
2. According to HT Mazumdar "a group of individuals is said to belong to a race when all its members share in common certain

significant physical traits that are transmitted biologically through the mechanism of heredity."
3. Horton and Hunt define race "as a group of people somewhat different from other groups in a combination of inherited physical characteristics, but race is also substantially determined by popular social definition."
4. According to Biesanz, "race is a large group of people distinguished by inherited physical differences."

Thus, race is a group of people having certain genetically transmitted characteristics, which vary within a certain range and differentiate them from other groups of people.

## ■ DETERMINANTS OF RACE

Race is determined on the basis of physical characteristics, which can be broadly of two types
1. Indefinite physical traits
2. Definite physical traits

*Indefinite Physical Traits*—Indefinite physical traits are those traits, which cannot be measured like the color of the skin, color and texture of the hair, structure and color of the eyes.

*Definite Physical Traits*—Definite Physical traits are those traits which can be measured like stature, structure of the head, structure of the nose, blood-group, length of the hands and feet and perimeter of the chest.

Though races are determined on the basis of the above mentioned traits, it is not possible to find all the traits of one race in all the people. Today, there is no pure race in the world because of the intermixing of people. Race has sociological significance also. The concept of race gives rise to the feelings of superiority and inferiority among the people. Human beings have different cultures and physiological characteristics. Usually, they tend to marry within their own group. This leads to a "we feeling" among them, which in turn gives rise to social consciousness. The idea of race has a direct and strong influence on the behavior of the people.

Anthropologists have grouped human beings into three major races. This classification is based on the theory that each race has certain specific physical traits. But the physical traits cannot be taken into consideration any longer according to modern theorists. This

is because the physical traits have no longer remained the same due to the interbreeding of races and also due to the effect of the environment like climate effecting the physical traits. Thus, the concept of a "pure" race is a myth. For theoretical purposes, the races may be studied as the following.
1. *The Caucasoid Race*—Which include most people of Europe, the Middle East and India.
2. *The Mongoloid Race*—Which include most Japanese, Chinese, Nepalese, Koreans, Vietnamese. The important races in this category are:
   a. *Asian Mongol*—Found in China, Japan and East India.
   b. *Micronesian Polynesian*—Found in the eastern islands of Melanesia.
3. *The Negroid Race*—Which include black African people and the American Negroes and their descendants. They are found in Africa. These include the following races.
   a. *Negro*—Found in Africa.
   b. *Far Eastern Pygmy*—Found in Andaman and Philippines.
   c. *Melanesian*—Found in South Pacific Islands.
   d. *Bushman and Holtentits*—Found in Kalahari Desert of Africa.
4. *Australoid*—Found in Australia.

## ■ RACES IN INDIA

According to Sir Herbert Risley, India has some of the following races.
a. *Pre-Dravidian type*—like the primitive tribes of the hills and jungles, such as the Bhils.
b. *The Dravidian type*—living in the South Peninsula.
c. *The Indo-Aryan type*—living in Kashmir, Punjab and Rajputana.
d. *The Aryo-Dravidian Type*—living in the Gangetic valley.
e. *The Cytho-Dravidian Type*—living in the east of Indus.
f. *The Mongoloid Type*—found in Assam and the foothills of the eastern Himalayas.
g. The Mongoloid Dravidian type.

According to JH Hutton, the Negrito races were probably the original occupants of India. Then came the Proto-australoids, followed by the Mediterranean race. The Alpine race entered India during the 4th century BC Finally by about 1500 BC the Indo-Aryan race entered India. Today in the modern world, there has been almost a complete mixing of various human groups and a pure race cannot exist.

### POINTS TO NOTE
1. Meaning–definition–determinations of race.
2. Types of races in India.

### NURSING IMPLICATIONS
Race like caste and class is a form of social stratification which is based on physical characteristics of the people.

### QUESTIONS
1. Meaning of race.
2. Define race. Give a brief account of the different races and their features.
3. What are the determinants of race?
4. Give a brief account of the races in India.

# CHAPTER 12

# Population

- Society and population
- Population distribution in India—demographic characteristics
- Malthusian theory
- Population explosion in India
- Causes and consequences of over population
- Population control measures

## ■ SOCIETY AND POPULATION

The number of people living in a particular geographical area is called as population. The scientific study of populations is known as demography. Demography studies the number of people living in a particular area, the changes that have taken place in the population over the last few years and to estimate the future trends on this basis, the composition of the population and the distribution of population in space. It deals with the demographic processes like fertility, mortality, marriage, migration and social mobility. These processes influence the population of a particular area.

These factors are also very important from the Sociological point of view as they help to understand the society in a better way. Demography studies the social factors, which have an influence on the population. The demographic processes are to a great extent socially determined. The growth of population is a social phenomenon and the characteristics of the population like age, sex, literacy, religion, occupation, marital patterns, etc. are socially important.

Human beings being social and cultural, the society cannot exist without socio-cultural interaction. Population trends are dependant upon societal factors. Therefore, there has to be a balance between them like the size of the population and the food supply or relation between nutrition and health. Only then the social order of the society can be maintained. Thus, there has to be an adjustment between the rate of population growth and the social conditions.

## Demographic Cycle

The history of the world population since 1650 suggests that there is a demographic cycle of five stages through which any nation passes. This is dependent upon the demographic processes of birth rates and death rates or fertility rates and mortality rates.

1. *First Stage*—This stage is characterized by a high birth rate and high death rate, resulting in the population remaining the same as the birth rates and the death rates balance each other. India was in this stage till 1920.
2. *Second Stage*—The death rate begins to fall while the birth rate remains the same. As a result, there is an increase in the population.
3. *Third Stage*—The death rate declines still further and the birth rate also tends to fall. The population continues to grow because the births exceed deaths.
4. *Fourth Stage*—In this stage, there is a low birth rate and a low death rate. The result is that the population remains the same.
5. *Fifth Stage*—The growth of the population begins to decline because the birth rate is lower than the death rate.

## ■ DISTRIBUTION OF POPULATION

The population of the earth is not evenly distributed in the various parts of the world. Some areas of the world are densely populated while some are very thinly populated. The density of population is defined as the number of persons living in per square area of land. This density of population in an area is dependent on a number of factors like climate, soil fertility, surface area, stage of economic development, etc. The densely settled areas of the world are the regions of Southern China, India, Europe and Eastern United States. The thinly populated areas are Siberia, Western United States, Australia, Africa, Canada and Polar regions. Asia, the largest continent has more than half the population of the world.

### Population Distribution in India

India is the second most populous country in the world, next to China. The Indian population has been growing at a rapid rate since 1920. The distribution of population in the States is very much uneven. The density of population has also been increasing along with the increase in population. It is defined as the number of people living in a per square area of land. The density of population is also unevenly distributed in the different states. Population of India is concentrated in a few states. The sex-composition of the population from the census figures also show that there is a successive decline in the sex-ratios of the population. Sex-ratio is the number of females per thousand males. Sex-composition is affected by the differentials in mortality conditions of males and females, sex-selective migration and sex-ratio at birth.

### Age-Pyramid or Age Distribution

The age-distribution of the Indian population, when diagrammatically shown, is in the form of a pyramid, which is typical of underdevelopment countries. It has a broad base and a tapering top. This is because of the high birth rate. The dependency population ratio in such cases is very high i.e. the children below 14 years of age and the elders above 65 years of age are more in number than the economically productive age group.

## ■ MALTHUSIAN THEORY OF POPULATION

Malthus, an English Economist, viewed the growth of population as a tragedy. In his first Essay on Population in 1798, he wrote "Population, when unchecked, increases in a geometrical ratio. Subsistence increases in an arithmetical ratio." According to him, the population would grow at a very fast rate, while the food would not increase at the same rate. Thus, an imbalance is created, which leads to overpopulation.

Malthus saw mankind doomed in huge, unless the growth of population was checked. He said that natural calamities like famine, diseases, war, would increase the death rate and bring about a short period equilibrium between population and food supply, which is disturbed sooner or later. These are the positive checks. He also advocated certain preventive checks like late marriage, moral restraint, artificial restraints, which can restrain the population from growing faster than subsistence.

## ■ POPULATION EXPLOSION IN INDIA

India is one of the most densely populated countries in the world. It is the second largest populated country in the world. It is overpopulated meaning too many people in relation to the sum of all kinds of resources. This growth of population is affecting the economic progress and development of the country. The census figures show an abnormal growth of population, especially since 1921, which can be called as the population explosion. India has 15% of the world population, but has only 2% of the world's land.

## Causes for the Rapid Growth of Population in India

Some of the causes for the growth of population in India are the following:
1. Decline in death rates due to progress in medicine.
2. Birth rates are higher than death rates.
3. Advancement in science and technology improvement in medicine and health facilities.
4. Universality of marriage and early marriage, resulting in high fertility and large families.
5. Indians are superstitions, fatalistic, prejudiced and ignorant.
6. The poor and agricultural families prefer to have more number of children for it would mean more number of working hands and more family income.
7. The high rate of illiteracy and ignorance among the people, combined with high infant morbidity and mortality rates also leads to high birth rate.
8. Lack of leisure-time activities, unemployment and poverty, industrialization, urbanization and migration are some of the factors contributing to high birth rate among the Indian population.

## ▪ EVIL EFFECTS OR CONSEQUENCES OF OVER-POPULATION

The overpopulation in India is a major problem for the country. Some of the effects or consequences of the rapid growth of population in India are the following:
1. *Population Growth and Development*—The high rate of growth of population hinders the progress and development of the economy. There is a heavy pressure on land and the natural resources become scarce in relation to the population and its consumption. Problem of unemployment and poverty increases.

These problems lead to a low standard of living and prevents economic growth.

2. *Food Problem*—The food production is not in proportion to the rapid rise of population in the country, which leads to food shortage and food problems. As a result, the people may suffer from malnutrition or may not get the proper daily requirement of food.
3. *Ill Health*—Unemployment coupled with poverty and malnutrition, effects the health of the population. The medical facilities like hospitals, doctors and paramedical staff are not sufficient for the growing population. Thus, there are a number of people affected both physically and mentally. It is observed that the number of people suffering from ill-health has been increasing in India, in spite of the advancement in medicine.
4. *Housing Problem*—The housing facilities are not enough for the growing population. People do not have the basic necessity of a proper shelter. The growth of slums, especially in the cities is an outcome of the rapid growth of population. People live in congested, ill-ventilated and poorly lighted houses, with unsanitary and unhygienic conditions, leading to health problems.
5. *Educational Facilities*—The educational facilities are not sufficient for the growing population. Thus illiteracy is very high.
6. *Low Standard of Living*—The economic growth is affected due to the increasing population. The rate of growth of national income, as well as the per capita income slows down, resulting in a low standard of living.

## Need for Population Control

The rapid growth of population in India is one of the major social problems, which needs immediate attention. The problem can be solved by taking up some measures to bring down the birth rates.

*Family Planning*—India is one of the first countries to adopt family planning as an official program in 1952. In 1977, it came to be called as "Family welfare". Family planning means planned parenthood i.e. conscious family limitation. It means having babies by choice and not by chance or God's will. Family planning is a way of thinking and living that is adopted voluntarily, on the basis of knowledge, attitudes and responsible decisions by individuals and couples, to promote the health and welfare of the family and thereby contribute effectively to the social development of the country. It refers to the practices that help individuals or couples to attain certain objectives like avoiding unwanted births or regulate the spacing of children or to determine the number of children in the family. The United Nations Conference on Human Rights at Teheran in 1968 and the Bucharest Conference on World Population held in August 1974 recognized family planning as a basic human right. Thus, during the past few years, family planning has emerged to the focus of international concern as a basic human right and as a component of family health and social welfare.

### POINTS TO NOTE
1. Demographic concept of population.
2. Processes of fertility, mortality, marriage, migration and social mobility. Influencing the population in a particular area.
3. Demographic cycle–population distribution in India.
4. Age pyramid or age distribution.
5. Malthusian theory of population.
6. Population explosion or over population in India. Its evil effects or consequences especially on health.
7. Need for population control and population education.

### NURSING IMPLICATIONS
Nurse has an important role as a population educator in case of over population in countries like India where illiteracy and ignorance is very high. The nurse can bring the awareness among the people about the high rate of growth of population, its health consequences and the need for population control.

### QUESTIONS
1. Define:
   a. Malthusian theory of population
   b. Population density
   c. Population explosion
   d. Age pyramid
2. Explain the causes of overpopulation.
3. What are the social consequences of population explosion?
4. Explain the role of the nurse in population education.
5. What are the effects of overpopulation on health?

# CHAPTER 13

# Social Control

- Norms and value
- Folkways and mores
- Customs, law and fashion
- Religion and public opinion
- Education, religion, coercion

## ■ MEANING

EA Ross was the first American sociologist to deal with the concept of social control in his book "Social Control" published in 1901. He was the first to use the concept in sociological discussion. Later on CH Colley and WG Sumner made important contributions to the development of this concept and understanding its nature and effects.

The peace and order of the society has to be maintained for the individuals to live in it. Society is a system of social relationships. It is the society, which is responsible for maintaining the social organization. The society therefore has to exercise control over the individual in order to exist and progress. This has been termed by sociologists as "social control". Social control is an influence, exerted by the society over the individual for promoting the welfare of the group as a whole. It is a system by which the society makes the individual to confirm to the approved patterns of the society through various agencies in the society. Social control has a specific aim or goal. The individual is made conscious of others and their interests and therefore follows the standard behavior patterns of the society.

## ■ DEFINITIONS

1. According to EA Ross, who was the first sociologist to use term, "social control refers to a system of devices whereby society

brings its members into conformity with the accepted standards of behavior."
2. Social control has been defined by Mac Iver and Page as "the way in which the entire social order coheres and maintains itself - how it operates as whole as a changing equilibrium."
3. Landis defines social control as "a social process by which the individual is made group-responsive and by which the social organization is built and maintained."
4. According to Ogburn and Nimkoff, social control is "the patterns of pressure, which a society exerts to maintain order and established rules."
5. Manheim defines social control as "the sum of those methods by which a society tries to influence human behavior to maintain given order."
6. GA Lundberg and others have defined social control as designating "those social behaviors, which influence individuals or groups towards conformity to established or desired norms."
7. Roucek has used the term social control for "those processes and agencies, planned or unplanned, by which individuals are taught, persuaded or compelled to confirm to the usages and life values of groups."
8. Kimball Young defines social control as "the use of coercion, force, restraint, suggestion or persuasion of one group over another or of a group over its members or of persons over others to enforce the prescribed rules of the game."

From the above definitions, it is clear that social control is a way of maintaining the peace and order of the society and the welfare of the group as a whole by the society through various mechanisms. Social control directs or guides the human behvior into socially desired goals. It operates on these levels- group over group, group over its members and individuals over their follows. In this way, social control brings about social conformity, social solidarity and assures the continuity of the group or society.

## ■ TYPES OF SOCIAL CONTROL

There are different ways of achieving social control in the society. Different sociologists have given different types of social control based on various factors. Karl Manheim classified social control as direct and indirect. Kimball Young classified it as positive and negative social control. According to Hayes, social control may be through sanction or through socialization and education. But most general type of classification of social control is on the basis of the means of social control that are employed. They are formal control and informal control.

1. *Informal Social Control*—Informal social controls are those controls, which grow on their own, when people continue to follow a set of behavior patterns. They are not specially made by man. Man learns many of these behavior patterns through the process of socialization. They become deep-rooted with the people and they follow them without any physical enforcement. There is no strong sanction or force behind them. But the people continue to follow them. These have a strong control in smaller and simpler societies. As the societies become complex and modern, they become less important for the individual. Hence, people may not observe them or they may go against them. Some of the informal social controls operating in the society are in the form of customs, traditions, folkways, mores, religion, ridicule, gossip, resentment, public opinion, etc. These are more effective in primary groups, which are small in size and have a personal relationship like the family, neighborhood, etc.

2. *Formal Social Control*—Formal social controls are specifically and deliberately created by man for controlling the behavior patterns of the individuals. As the society becomes more modern and complex in nature, the informal means of social control are not sufficient to maintain the order and harmony of the society. Different kinds of political, economic and cultural and other associations and institutions emerge in the society. The growth of secondary groups in the society, which may be very large in size and number in the modern complex societies, necessitates the formulation of norms and rules to control the behavior of its members. These are the formal social controls, which are in the form of laws, police, army, military, etc. The formal controls have a strong sanction or force behind them like punishment. If the members do not follow them, they would be punished, which would depend upon the nature and type of violation. They become

a necessity in the modern complex societies where the interaction is mostly impersonal in nature.

## NORMS AND VALUES

### Social Norms or Group Norms

*Meaning*

Man being a social animal cannot live alone. He has to have relationships with other human beings. These relationships give rise to behavior patterns, which have to be controlled. Social norms are the standard expected and accepted behavior patterns of the society. The social order of the society is maintained through these social norms. The concept of the "social norms" is important in Sociology because they form the foundation of the social structure of the society. They are also known as standards of group behavior.

Social norms are very important for the society. It is impossible to imagine a normless society. Norms help the individuals to have self-control and thereby help in maintaining the social order. They give cohesion to the society. Norms have a sanction or force behind them, which could be in the form of punishment or rewards, due to which individuals follow them or conform to them. Conformity to the norms is normal and is achieved through the process of socialization. The individual, who is socialized, feels the compulsion to follow them. Further, there would be disapproval of his behavior if he violates them. Thus, the internalization of the norms and the external sanctions, play an important role in bringing about conformity to the norms.

*Definition*

1. Broom and Selznick define norms as "the blueprints for behavior setting limits within which individuals may seek alternate ways to achieve their goals."
2. Robert Bierstedt says that "a norm is a rule or standard that governs our conduct in the social situations in which we participate."
3. According to Harry M Johnson "a norm is an abstract pattern held in the mind that sets certain limits for behavior."

4. GR Leslie, RF Larson and BL Gorman opine that "social norms are rules developed by a group of people that specify how people must, should, may, should not and must not behave in various situations."

Thus, in general, it can be said that norms are rules and regulations that groups follow. They are the means through which values are expressed in the behaviors of the members.

## Social Values

### Meaning

Social values are the measurers of the goodness or desirability, which act as guidelines for the behavior of the people. They are important for an organized social life. Social values are the abstract ideals or sentiments, regulating the individual's thinking and behavior patterns. They become a part of the culture of the society through the process of socialization. Social values, social norms and institutions explain the way in which the social processes operate in a given society.

Thus, they help in maintaining the social order and stability of the society by acting as social controls. Individuals use values as criteria for assessing their daily lives, arranging the priorities, measuring their pleasures and pains, choosing between alternative causes of action. The values of a society therefore provide the goals or ends for its members to aim for.

### Definition

1. According to Harry M Johnson "values are general standards and may be regarded as higher order norms."
2. GR Leslie and others define it as "group conceptions of the relative desirability of things."

Thus social values are the wide range of ideas about the ends that men should pursue in their life.

## Agencies of Social Control

Society or group maintain social control by creating their own agencies which may be formal and informal. Agencies like law, education, physical coercion and codes are formal in nature while agencies like folkways, mores, customs and traditions, religion, etc., are informal controls used by the society for this purpose.

Some of the important informal agencies of social control are the following

## Religion

Religion is a belief system. It is the belief in some super-natural power, which is called as God. It is mans relationship with God, which makes him good, obedient and helpful to others. Thus, it regulates the behavior of man and enforces discipline. In this way, it acts as an informal means of social control. Religion teaches the values of life through the agencies of socialization like family, school, etc.

## ■ FOLKWAYS AND MORES

### Folkways

#### Meaning

Folkways are the informal type of social controls. "Folkways" refer to the "ways of the folk" i.e. the ways of the people. This term was first used by WG Sumner in his sociological classic "Folkways" in 1906, who studied and analyzed culture and its implications. Sumner conceived culture in terms of folkways and mores. Folkways are the recognized ways of behavior and acting in the society, which arise automatically within a group to meet the problems of social living. They are the repetitive petty acts of the people, like how to eat, how to dress, how to speak, how to greet each other, etc. It is passed on form one generation to the next and becomes one of the ways of the group- of the folk - hence a "Folkway". They are collective, unconscious modes of behavior that are believed to ensure the survival of the group. Folkways include the different ways of behavior that men have evolved for their social living. They are the customs and usages which have been passed on form generation to generation and to which new elements are added according to the changing needs and times. They represent man's unique means of adapting himself to his environment.

## Definition

1. Mac Iver and Page defined folkways as "the recognized and accepted ways of behaving in the society."
2. According to Horton and Hunt folkways are "simply the customary, normal and habitual ways of doing things."
3. Merill and Eldridge say that folkways are "literally the ways of the folk i.e., social habits or group expectations that have arisen in the daily life of the group."
4. Gillin and Gillin define folkways as "the behavior patterns of everyday life, which generally arise unconsciously in a group."

## Characteristics of Folkways

Some of the important characteristics of folkways are:
1. *Spontaneous Origin*—Folkways are not deliberately designed. They are spontaneous and develop out of experience.
2. *Approved Behavior*—Folkways are the behavior patterns that have been approved and recognized by the group to which they relate.
3. *Distinctiveness*—Each group develops its own folkways that differs from society to society and from group to group. Thus, there are a variety of folkways.
4. *Heredity*—Folkways are passed on from generation to generation. They are learnt through the process of socialization as a part of the culture of the group. Folkways become a habit for the individuals and the group.
5. *Folkways keep Changing*—Folkways do not remain the same. They keep changing from time to time, to suit the social changes and the social conditions.
6. *Sanction of Folkways*—The sanction or force behind folkways is informal. Hence, the punishment for the violation of the folkways is not very severe. It may be in the form of gossip or ridicule or criticism.

## Mores

"Mores" or "morals" like folkway are also informal type of social controls. But they are stronger than the folkways because the sanction or force behind them is stronger. The violation of a more has a stronger punishment behind it. WG Sumner used the term "mores" to those folkways, which are considered by the group to be of great significance and therefore indispensable for the group welfare. The term "mores" is derived from the Latin word "mos" which stands for "customs". When folkways act as regulators of behavior then they become "mores". They imply a value judgment about the folkways. "Mores" have the element of truth and right. They express the group sense of what is fitting, right and conducive to social welfare and the group. Hence, they become more compulsive in nature.

"Mores" may be positive or negative. Positive "mores" prescribe behavior patterns while negative "mores" prohibit certain behavior patterns. Every group has its own "mores". They help the individual to identify themselves with the group and bring about a solidarity and harmony of group. There are "mores" for each sex, for all ages, for all classes, for all families and so on.

## Definitions

1. Mac Iver and Page have said that "when the folkways have added to them conceptions of group welfare, standards of right and wrong, they are converted into "mores."
2. Gillin and Gillin had defined "mores" as "those customs and group routines, which are thought by the members of the society to be necessary to the group existence."

From the above discussion, it is clear that "mores" determine our conceptions of what is proper or improper, right or wrong. They are not the same everywhere. There is a great variation in the "mores" from group to group. For example, one group allows polygyny while another group may condemn it. Therefore, "mores" may appear proper and right for one group and improper for another group. Also, "mores" keep changing from time to time. "Mores" can make some thing appear right at one time and wrong at another time like the changing dress patterns of the Indian women. Thus, "mores" play an important role for the individual and for the society. Accordingly, "mores" have the important function of determining much of the individual behavior of identifying the individual with the group and finally acting as the guardians of solidarity.

## Distinction between Folkways and Mores

A distinction has been made between folkways and "mores". According to WG Sumner, when the folkways "take on a philosophy

of right living and a life policy of welfare, then they become "mores'."
A distinction between folkways and "mores" can be made in the following ways:

1. Folkways are more general and wider in nature whereas "mores" are more particular in character.
2. Mores have a value judgment about the folkways while folkways do not imply any value judgment.
3. "Mores" are more effective in regulating the behavior of the people. They are stronger than the folkways because they have a stronger sanction behind them. Folkways are not very effective in regulating people's behavior because they do not have a very strong force behind them. Folkways are the recognized ways of behaving and acting.
4. The convictions of right and wrong arise out of the "mores" and not out of the folkways.
5. "Mores" are deeply rooted in the society and therefore, do not change easily whereas folkways are less deeply rooted in society and therefore, change more rapidly.
6. Violation of the "mores" is a danger to the rights of others but violation of the folkways does not effect anyone.

## Customs

Custom is a social phenomenon, the origin of which is obscure. Customs are certain ways of acting which are passed on from generation to generation. These have a social significance because customs are socially recognized and customs are normative in nature. They regulate the life of the individual and the groups of individuals. Man learns them from his childhood and follows them as a matter of habit. They act as a storehouse of human experiences determining and controlling human behavior. Thus, they are able to maintain the social order and peace in the society.

## Definition

1. According to Ginsberg "custom is not merely a prevailing habit, but also a rule or norm of action."
2. Mac Iver defines it as "a group procedure that has gradually emerged, without express enactment, without any constitute authority to declare it, to apply it, to safeguard it."

3. Kingsley Davis is of the opinion that "custom" is closer to 'folkways' than to "mores", but it tends to convey the traditional, automatic and mass character of both of them."
4. According to Lundberg, customs are "those folkways that persist over relatively long periods of time so as to attain the degree of formal recognition and so as to be passed down from one generation to another."

Thus, customs are the long-established habits and usages of the people. Wherever there is a widespread habit, there is a corresponding custom.

## THE SOCIAL ROLE OF CUSTOM

Customs play an important part in the life of the individual, as well as the society. Customs are the informal social controls of the society. Customs acted as very strong controls in the primitive society but in the modem complex societies, they are loosing their hold over the people.

Custom regulates social life. It is an important means of controlling social behavior. Customs are accepted and followed by the society because they have been followed in the past. They are very powerful and no one can escape their range. Customs regulate social life to a great extent because many of the daily activities of man like dressing speaking, eating, worshipping, celebrations, etc., are all controlled by customs. They are the habits and usages of the people, which have persisted for a long time and which have been passed on from one generation to another. Customs are obeyed more spontaneously and unconsciously. Thus, custom is the repository of social heritage. It preserves our culture.

Customs help to mould the personality of the individual. They are learnt by the individual in the process of his growth and socialization, which goes on from the time of his birth till his death. He is controlled by them throughout his life. Thus, they mould his attitudes and ideas, thereby acting as informal means of social controls.

Customs are universal. They are accepted and followed by the society because they have been followed in the past. There is no constituted authority to declare, to apply or safeguard them. In this way, they are able to regulate social life.

Customs are the savers of energy. Many of the daily activities of man like the ways of dressing, speaking, eating, worshipping, etc., are regulated by customs. People do not have to think about these daily activities. They just follow them as a matter of habit, which saves them the time and energy in their daily activities. People therefore, confirm to them spontaneously and unconsciously. Customs therefore become basic to collective life and held so sacred that any violation of them is regarded not only as a crime but also a sacrilege.

Some of the important agencies of formal social control are the following:

## Laws

Laws are the most powerful formal means of social control. As the societies grow and become more complex, the informal means of social control like the customs, mores, folkways, etc., are not enough to control the people's behavior and maintain the social order and peace in the society. Thus, laws had to be enacted by the state to control the individuals.

Laws appear only in societies with a political organization. Law need a special agency or a machinery to frame them and enforce them. Laws are clearly written down, which are equally applicable to all without any exception. They also prescribe the punishments for violation of the laws, which may range from a simple fine to a severe punishment like imprisonment or life sentence. Laws are enforced with the help of the police, the court and sometimes the armed forces.

## Definitions

1. Mac Iver and Page define law as "the body of rules, which are recognized, interpreted and applied to particular situations by the courts of the state."
2. According to Sumner, "laws are the codified "mores".
3. According to Duguit laws are "the rules of conduct, which normal men know that they must observe in order to preserve and promote the benefits derived from life in the society."
4. JS Roucek is of the opinion that "laws are a form of social rule emanating from political agencies."

## Characteristics of Laws

From the above discussion, the important characteristics of laws are the following:
1. Laws are the general conditions of human activity prescribed by the state for its members.
2. Law is law only if it is enacted by a proper lawmaking authority. It is a product of conscious thought, planning and deliberate formulation.
3. Law is definite, clear and precise.
4. Law applies equally without exception in identical circumstances.
5. Violation of law is followed by penalties determined by the authority of the state.

## Differences between Custom and Law

In order to have an understanding of the nature of law and custom, it is important to understand the differences between the two. Some of the important differences between the two are the following:
1. Law is specially enacted by a proper lawmaking authority. It is consciously and deliberately thought and planned for the general conditions of human activity. Law is prescribed by the state for its members whereas customs just grow in the society. They are certain ways of acting, which are passed on from generation to generation.
2. Law is definite, specific and clear. It is enacted by a proper lawmaking authority while customs are not definite and clear.
3. Law needs a special agency for enforcement. The violation of law is followed by penalties determined by the authority of the state. Custom does not need any agency for enforcement. Also, there is no penalty attached to the violation of a custom.
4. Law can be changed or abolished only by the lawmaking authority whereas customs may fade or disappear without any formal abolition.
5. Law is more flexible and adaptable than custom. Law can be introduced, amended or abolished with relative ease whereas customs cannot be easily changed because they are comparatively fixed and permanent.

6. Law is more idealistic than custom. It is deliberately enacted with certain aims. Therefore, law is more idealistic but custom is a practice, which is concerned with the daily routine of life.
7. Law is concerned with important aspects of the life of the society while custom is concerned with ordinary, familiar and daily aspects of life.

Inspite of the differences cited above, it can be said that law and custom supplement and complement each other.

### Education

Education is a process of socialization through which the social heritage of a group is passed on from one generation to the next. It prepares the individuals for his future. It molds the individual's personality. It modifies the thoughts, feelings and action it regulates the behavior of people and thus act as an agent of social control it contributes to the regulation of conduct in the early socialization of the child. It must be used for making a good society. It is through education that the new generation learns the social norms and the penalties for violating them with education, social controls become normal. Hence, education is necessary condition for proper exercise of social control.

### Coercion

The use of coercion or force is another means to achieve social control in the society. It is use to stop or control a work or an action. It is an extreme form of violence which the state uses to control anti-social activities and maintain social order and peace.

### ■ FASHION

Fashion means "style". It is an important informal means of social control. Fashion determines the speech, opinion, belief, recreation, dress, music, art and literature, etc. It can be observed in all fields of life. Fashion is one of the most temporary or short–lived forms of social control. It keeps changing very often. Fashion is a behavior pattern, which is generally started by people belonging to a higher class. It is then imitated by others. Those who start with a fashion become the "role-model" for the others to imitate. Thus, Gabriel Trade defined it as the "imitation of contemporaries". Herbert Spencer regarded it as "a leveler of custom".

## Characteristics of Fashion

1. *Fashion is a Group Choice*—Fashion is not an individual choice. It is a group choice, i.e. it is a behavior pattern adopted by a number of people.
2. *Fashion Changes Rapidly*—Fashions keep changing from time to time and place to place. If they continue to remain in the society for a long time, they may become "folkways" or a "more".
3. *Fashion does not Need Utility*—Element of utility may or may not be there in fashion. Every fashion need not have any utility or purpose.
4. *Fashions are All-Pervasive*—Fashions can be observed in different areas of social life like dress, speech, foods, beliefs, opinions, art, literature, music, etc.

## Differences between Custom and Fashion

1. Custom is enduring whereas fashion keeps changing. Custom continues to remain in the society since the people keep following it through the generations. Fashion is short-lived.
2. Custom is a social habit, which is passed on from generation to generation. It grows by itself. Therefore, it is spontaneous while fashion is created by man. It is artificial.
3. Custom is concerned with the society whereas fashion concerns the individual, i.e. custom is followed by all the members of a community, which creates a social bond between them but fashion is started by somebody and others may or may not adopt it.
4. Custom is concerned with important matters of social life while fashion is concerned with trivial aspects of the life of the individual.
5. Fashion grows when custom breaks off in the society. Fashion is more common in the modem society than in the traditional society because custom may start losing its importance in the modem society.

## ■ THE SOCIAL ROLE OF FASHION IN THE MODERN SOCIETY

Fashion is a transitory accepted change. It is short-lived but has an important social role to play especially in the modem society.
1. Fashion satisfies two strong desires of man i.e. the demand for novelty and the demand for conformity. Man yearns for something new for a variety. Fashion satisfies this desire of man, which is necessary for his living in the society. Thus, it succeeds in accommodating this desire to the rule of conformity.
2. Fashion facilitates social change by providing a transitional stage from one custom to another. It tries to bring about a change in the customs and beliefs. The "cake of customs", which is hard to break is modified by fashion.
3. Fashion generally originates in the higher classes of the society, whose prestige is enhanced. This is imitated by other classes in the society.

Thus, fashion plays an important role in simultaneously satisfying the contrary desires for novelty and for conformity. It controls the individuals thoughts, ideas, attitudes and behavior.

> **POINTS TO NOTE**
>
> 1. Social control–meaning–types–formal and informal means of social control.
> 2. Different types of social control.
>    a. Norms and values.
>    b. Folk ways and mores.
>    c. Customs, laws and fashion.
>    d. Religion and education.
>    e. Coercion

> **NURSING IMPLICATIONS**
>
> Social controls are ways and means of maintaining peace and order of the society for the welfare of the people. The different types both formal and informal controls help to control behavior pattern of the people. It helps the nurse to use these means to control and understand the behavior of the patients.

## QUESTIONS

1. Define:
   a. Social control
   b. Formal means of social control
   c. Informal means of social control
   d. Fashion
   e. Folkways
   f. Customs
   g. Laws
   h. Mores
   i. Norms
   j. Values
   k. Education
   l. Coercion
   m. Religion
2. Differentiate between:
   a. Folkways and mores.
   b. Custom and law.
3. What is social control? Enumerate the important social control measures in the society.
4. Describe the social control measures in the society.
5. Explain how the agencies of social control help in regulating human behavior.

# CHAPTER 14

# Social Problems

- Social Disorganization-characteristics and causes
  - Poverty
  - Beggary
  - Alcoholism
- Social problems-meaning and classification
  - Control and planning
  a. Major social problem poverty and unemployment
    - Housing
    - Illiteracy
    - Food supplies
    - Prostitution
    - Rights of women and children-gathery or alcoholism
- Vulnerable groups
  - Elderly
  - Handicapped
  - Minority and other marginalized groups
  - Child labor - child abuse
  - Delinquency and crime
  - Substance abuse
  - HIV/AIDS
- Social Welfare Programs in India

## ■ SOCIAL DISORGANIZATION

Society has been defined as the system or web of social relations. These social relationships give rise to social behaviors, social groups, social institutions, etc., which make up the social structure of the society. When the social relationships, making up the social structure of the society get disintegrated, there is social disorganization.

Society, being understood as a system of social relationships between individuals, is controlled and regulated by institutions and associations. Social controls like folkways, mores, customs, laws, beliefs, attitudes, values and ideals, maintain the equilibrium between the various elements of the society. When the equilibrium between the different elements of society changes, a breakdown of the social structure of the society occurs, resulting in social disorganization. Emile Durkheim therefore defined social disorganization as "a state of disequilibrium and a lack of social solidarity or consensus among the members of a society." According to Ogburn and Nimkoff social disorganization occurs "when the harmonious relationship between the various parts of culture is disturbed."

## Characteristics

Some of the important characteristics of social disorganization are the following:

1. *Conflict of mores and institutions*—Changes in the traditional mores and institutions of the society come into conflict with the new ones, destroying the consensus of the society. This disrupts the organization and social disorganization of the society sets in. For example, differences of opinion with respect to some social laws and social institutions like divorce, caste system, untouchability, widow remarriage, love marriage, family system, etc. in the Indian society.
2. *Transfer of functions from one group to another*—Society is dynamic. Therefore, as changes take place in the society, the predetermined functions of the groups also change and are transferred to another group leading to disorganization. For example, many of the traditional functions of the family have been taken over by other agencies like the nurseries, schools, hospitals, clubs, etc.
3. *Individuation*—In the modern age, individualism has increased, where the individual makes his own decisions regarding important aspects of his life like his marriage and family, occupation, moral conduct, etc. This leads to a change in and diversification of social values.
4. *Changes in the role and status of the individuals*—Changes in the society effect a change in the role and status of the individuals. People begin to choose from among the different roles, which cause disequilibrium leading to a social disorganization. Change in the status of woman in India has lead to the disorganization of the family.

From the above characteristics of social disorganization, it can be concluded that it is a process. Sociologists regard social disorganization as a natural process rather than a malady. The social consensus gets disturbed. It is an indication of the existence of disease or disruptive elements in the society. It can be known by its symptoms. Sociologists have listed different symptoms of social disorganization. Elliot and Merril have pointed out that social disorganization may be of three types, i.e. the disorganization of the individual, the family and the community. Among the symptoms of individual disorganization they include juvenile delinquency, different types of crime, insanity, drunkenness, suicide and prostitution. Among the symptoms of family disorganization they include divorce, illegitimate births, desertion and venereal diseases. Among the symptoms of community disorganization they include poverty, unemployment, crime and corruption. But no definite difference can be made among these three types of disorganization as they are all interdependent and one kind of social disorganization may lead to another.

## Causes

1. *Social Change*—Changes is the order of nature. Society is dynamic. The elements of the society are constantly changing like mores, customs, institutions, technology, culture, etc. With this change, the old elements come into conflict with the new ones, resulting in a disorder and there by a social disorganization.
2. *Cultural Factors*—Ogburn developed the concept of cultural-lag while studying social changes in the society. According to him, different aspects of culture change at different rates leading to a conflict between them. He differentiated between material and nonmaterial culture. In his study of social changes and social problems, Ogburn observed that the material culture change faster than the nonmaterial culture, causing a cultural-lag and producing a consequent social disorganization. According to him, social problems like unemployment, crime, poverty, family disorganization, labor problems, etc., are all due to irregular changes in culture.
3. *National Catastrophies*—According to Ogburn, ecological disturbances i.e. disturbances in the relationship of man to his environment also lead to social disorganization. For e.g., diseases, earthquakes, floods, etc., over which man has no control.

4. *War*—War causes confusion and disorder in the society because it leads to economic crisis and also tends to weaken the sexual ties as it affects the male-female ratio. Social values also get effected. For example, the value of the human life is reduced.
5. *Crisis*—Crisis is a condition, which disturbs the social order of the society by focusing upon a conflict situation. For example, an accident or the sudden death of a leader like Mahatma Gandhi.
6. *Change in Social Values*—Every society has its own social values. These act as social controls in the society. They maintain the order and organization of the society. These keep changing with time. The new values come into conflict with the old values resulting in social disorganization. Changes in the traditional values regarding the caste system or the traditional joint family in India have occurred, resulting in a conflict between the old and the new values. Thus, the process of social disorganization has occurred.

## SOCIAL PROBLEMS

It has been noted that social disorganization occurs when the equilibrium between the different elements of the society is disturbed. A social problem is said to exist when an individual or a group of individuals is disorganized. They are not functioning according to the norms of the society. Thus, social disorganization is always a result of some breakdown in the social organization. Social problems are the conditions threatening the well-being of the society.

Social problems are behavior patterns or conditions that are considered to be undesirable by a major part of the population in the society. A social problem according to Lundberg is "any deviant behavior like a disapproved direction." Social problems are subjective in nature. But there are some problems like poverty, unemployment, war, crime, etc., which are universal and permanent and are found in almost all societies.

Every social problem implies:
1. That something should be done to change the situation, which constitutes a problem.
2. That the existing social order has to be changed to solve the problem.
3. That the situation regarded as a problem is undesirable but not inevitable.

There are both individual and social problems. Individual problems become social problems when they effect a large portion of population and become a threat to the welfare and safety of the larger group. But all individual problems need not be social problems. Some social problems are public health problems like crime, divorce, housing growth of population, increased number of old people, poverty and diseases. Some social problems like alcoholism, venereal diseases, mental illness and drug addiction are also public health problem. No single cause can be pointed out for a social problem.

Harold A Phelps classified social problems as:
1. *Economic Problems*—poverty, unemployment and dependency.
2. *Biological Problems*—physical diseases and defects.
3. *Psychological Problems*—neurosis, psychosis, epilepsy, feeble-mindedness, suicide and alcoholism.
4. *Cultural Problems*—problems of the aged, the homeless, the widowed, divorced, illegitimacy, crime and juvenile delinquency.

# ■ MAJOR SOCIAL PROBLEMS

## Poverty

Poverty is one of the major social problems in countries like India. It is related to the problem of overpopulation and unemployment. It is a concept used with relation to richness, because there have always been the rich and the poor classes in the society. Poverty is a condition when an individual is not able to buy the basic necessities of life like food, shelter and clothing and there by not able to maintain himself and those dependent on him in good health. Poverty, coupled with unemployment are the two major social problems leading to sickness and disease and also personal, family and community disorganization.

Gillin and Gillin have defined poverty as "a condition in which a person either because of inadequate income or unwise expenditures does not maintain a scale of living high enough to provide for his mental and physical efficiency and to enable him and his natural dependents to function usually according to the standards of a society of which he is a member."

Poverty may be called as absolute poverty when an individual is not able to maintain himself and his family at a subsistence level i.e., when he is not able to buy the minimum subsistence requirement like food, clothing and shelter. It may be called as relative poverty when an individual is comparatively poor to individuals within his own group.

## Causes

1. Poverty of an individual may be due to the incapacity of the individual like hereditary weakness, physical and mental handicaps, attitudes towards work, etc.
2. Adverse physical and geographical conditions also lead to poverty like natural disasters – floods, earthquakes, drought, famine, etc., over which man does not have any control. Also poor natural resources and excessive dependence on nature may lead to poverty.
3. Changes in technology and the economic conditions like shortage of capital, unequal distribution of wealth, economic depression may result in poverty.
4. Poverty and educational levels are related. Lack of knowledge, laziness and idleness contribute to poverty. Also, spending beyond their means on festivals, marriages, religious ceremonies, etc. leads to a condition of poverty since they would not have the money to spend on the basic necessities of life.
5. Indulgence in some bad activities like drinking, prostitution, gambling may force an individual and his dependents to a state of poverty.
6. Uncontrolled reproduction leading to a large number of dependents per earning member, death of an earning member, calamities in the family, may also lead to poverty of the family.
7. Unemployment, unproductive hoarding, unwise economic policy, faulty educational system, inadequate housing, certain evil customs and practices, insufficient medical facilities, etc. are also responsible for reducing the efficiency of the individuals and increasing the poverty of a region.

## Remedial Measures

Poverty has been one of the major social problems in India. Therefore, after Independence, the government decided to have programs for the removal of poverty in the country. For this purpose, they started taking a number of measures, launched many schemes, programs and projects for the removal of poverty.

After Independence, the Indian Government setup the Planning Commission in 1950 and started the Five Year Plans for the development of the country. These plans mainly aimed at achieving self-reliance in agriculture, removing unemployment and achieving industrial progress, increasing the standard of living and the removal of poverty. A number of policies and programs were adopted by the government for this purpose. These are known as the Poverty Alleviation Programs (PAP). They aim at providing employment and improving the conditions of the poor. Some of the anti-poverty programs taken up by the government are Swarnjayanti Gram Swarojgar Yojna (SGSY), Jawahar Gram Samriddhi Yojna (JGSY), Prime Minister's Rojgar Yojana (PMRY), Swarnjayanti Shahari Rojgar Yojana (SJSRY), Employment Assurance Scheme (EAS), Pradhanamantri Gramoday Yojana (PMGY), Integrated Rural Development Program (IRDP), National Rural Employment Program (NREP) and Antyodaya Program. All these programs aim at creating wage employment for families below poverty line and improving the quality of life of the poor.

# UNEMPLOYMENT

Unemployment is a major social problem along with the problem of poverty in the Indian society. The problem of unemployment leads to the problem of poverty. This two problems go together in most societies. Therefore they called as the twin problem of the society. This is a serious problem in India which is due to the unprecedented growth of population. Unemployment can set to be a condition where the able-bodied and willing to work labor force are not gainfully employed. They are not able to find work unemployment can be of different type like seasonal unemployment, Agricultural unemployment, frictional and technological unemployment, industrial unemployment, cyclical unemployment, educational unemployment, voluntary unemployment, involuntary unemployment, under unemployment, open unemployment and disguised unemployment.

## Causes

There are a number of factor responsible for unemployment individual and social factors are responsible for unemployment.

Unemployment and poverty are inter-related. Unemployment may be the cause, of poverty or poverty may be the cause of unemployment. It is one of the most important causes of social disorganization. According to GR Madan there are two types of causes of unemployment.
1. Individual or personal factors.
2. External factors or technological and economic factors.

The individual or personal factors are age factor, vocational unfitness, illness or physical disabilities or incapabilities.

The external factors are increasing population, trade cycles, technological advancement like mechanization and automation, strikes and lockouts, slow rate of economic growth etc. Besides these, there are also other causes like unpreparedness to accept socially degrading jobs, defects in educational system, geographic immobility of workers, improper use of human resources and lack of encouragement for self-employment.

### Effects or Impact

Unemployment is lead to personal disorganization, family disorganization, social disorganization and economic losses. It become a socio-economic problem for the society. Some remedial measures like population control, promoting economic development and industrial development, educational reforms and vocational programs or training implemented through five year plans.

The twin problem of unemployment and poverty have an effect on the health of the individual as well as the members of his family since he will not be having the resources to maintain the health of the individuals as he may not be able to provide the basic necessities of life for his dependents.

## ■ BEGGARY

The twin problems of poverty and unemployment are associated with the problem of beggary. It is grave problem in under-developed and developing countries like India. Beggars are found wandering on the streets, public places, markets, temples, bus stands, railway stations, etc. It is a personal disorganization. A beggar is one who asks for alms or charity.

## Types

Dr Kumarappa has classified the beggars into the following types:
- Child beggars, who may be paid or unpaid assistants of the adult beggars.
- Physically disabled, chronically under nourished and those afflicted with diseases.
- Mentally disabled.
- Able bodied, who are lazy to work and earn their living.
- Religious mendicants in the form of *sadhus, sanyasis, fakirs* and others.
- Bogus mendicants, who are able-bodied individuals in the garb of *fakirs* or *sanyasis* and draw generosity of religious minded people.
- Tribal beggars who move from place to place singing and reciting local songs and begging.
- Hereditary beggars who are professional beggars.
- Infirm or old people.
- Seasonally unemployed individuals who migrate to larger cities in the off-season and live by begging.
- Permanently unemployed who are not able to find employment though they are ready to work, resort to begging.

## Causes

Beggary is a very complex individual and social problem which is a result of a number of causes. It is related to other social problem like poverty and unemployment, crippling diseases which may be physical or mental, lack provision for old age and social security, disintegration of the joint family, family disorganization like divorce, separation and religious sanctions, charity and public sympathy for mankind.

## Measures to Overcome Beggary

Most countries have prohibited beggary and declared it an offence. Inspite of it, it continues to be a major problem in developing countries like India. State intervention and legislation are necessary if the problems of beggary along with destitution and vagrancy have to be solved. Special acts have been passed in most of the states in

India to prohibit beggary in public places. There are rehabilitation centers established for beggars in the states wher they are provided with basic necessities of life. Besides these, some other measures that can be taken to lesson this problem are:
1. Old attitudes towards charity.
2. Giver of the charity should also be punished.
3. Provide alternate employment.
4. Social security services should be developed.
5. Different treatment has to be adjusted to the different categories of beggars.
6. Provide after-care and follow-up action.
7. Provision of sterilization of persons suffering from hereditary diseases.

## ILLITERACY

Education is one of the fundamental rights of the individual. The term "education" is derived from the Latin word "educare" meaning to "bring up" and "bring forth". It is a continuous process of learning for the individual. Education is a part of the socialization of the individual where he learns to behave according to the norms of the society. It is also an important way of transmitting the culture to the next generation. Thus, it is a deliberate process of training the individual to fulfill his basic needs and to develop his personality. Therefore, it is very important for the individual to be educated.

Education and literacy are related. Education is essential for the progress and development of the society. Illiteracy is the condition where an individual is not able to read and sign his name. Such individuals will live in poverty and have poor health.

Illiteracy is one of the basic causes of most of the social problems of the society. Unemployment and poverty are some of the consequences of illiteracy, which in turn results in bad living conditions due to ignorance of basic health and hygiene awareness.

With literacy, the understanding of the importance of health, sanitation and nutrition of their families is better thereby reducing the incidence of the preventable illness and death. There is also greater financial and social stability.

There are a number of reasons for illiteracy. It has been observed that in countries like India, the illiteracy is higher among the girls due to the gender bias. Also, the conditions of poverty and unemployment, force them to work. The quality of education may not be good, with a glaring lack of minimum facilities of teaching, good sanitation and hygiene. Diseases and pests spread easily.

## ▪ HOUSING

Housing, food, clothing, health care, education, etc. are the basic needs of the people in any society. The economic conditions of the individuals determine their capacity to possess the basic needs and necessities of life for a comfortable living. People who are unable to do this are physically weak and are not able to work efficiently, which in turn affects the progress of the society.

A minimum standard of housing is necessary to maintain the health of the population. In the poor countries, housing activities should be given importance. This will improve the quality of life, especially of the poorer sections of the society, which will help in the achievement of objectives of health, sanitation and education.

The problem of housing is very grave in India, both in the rural and urban areas. Housing conditions are no doubt improving in rural areas. For example, there are cemented houses, which are more airy and cleaner, with electricity and water facilities and sanitation is improving.

The major consequence of the problem of housing in urban areas is the growth of slums. The growth of slums is a peculiar feature of the unplanned growth of cities. The cities become centers of attraction for the people of smaller towns and villages. With increased migration from these areas to the cities, there is a high concentration of people in urban-industrial areas. It results in overcrowding, congestion, housing problems, growth of slums, lack of water facilities and sanitation, etc.

The people in slums live in very bad areas, where the minimum and basic facilities for a living are absent. They live in the most unhygienic conditions, which results in a number of health problems. Diseases spread in epidemic proportions. There is a scarcity of health and welfare services.

The houses in slums are unfit for human habitation. They are a centre of all kinds of anti-social activities and vices like gambling, prostitution, alcoholism, crime, juvenile delinquency, etc. Thus, the physical, mental and moral life of the people is in danger.

The policy planners and house building agencies should take up slum improvement programs with a multidimensional approach by taking into consideration various factors like the functional needs of the population, anticipated service facilities and the socioeconomic and cultural variations and needs of the population that has to be housed.

## ■ FOOD SUPPLIES

Food along with shelter and clothing is the basic need of man for his survival. Lack of proper food, result in problems of hunger and malnutrition. Malnutrition has been defined as "a pathological state resulting from a relative or absolute deficiency or excess of one or more essential nutrients." It is a manmade disease of the human societies. A number of factors like conditioning influences, cultural influences, socioeconomic factors, food production, health and other services are responsible for malnutrition.

Malnutrition is a major problem in most underdeveloped or developing countries due to the high rate of growth of population. In such countries, it is largely due to poverty, ignorance, insufficient education, lack of knowledge regarding the nutritive value of foods, inadequate sanitary environment, large family size, etc., which have a direct impact on the quality of life of the people.

Increased food production should lead to increased food consumption. But, this does not happen in most underdeveloped countries. The problem of hunger and malnutrition still continue to remain in the society. It is more of a problem of equitable distribution of food in accordance with the physiological needs.

It can be solved only by taking action simultaneously at various levels - family, community, national and international levels. This requires a coordinated approach by many disciplines - nutrition, food technology, health administration, health education, marketing etc. There has to be a comprehensive program of social development of the country with action to be taken at the family level, community level, national level and international level.

*At the Family Level*—At the family level, nutrition education will help in combating malnutrition. Other related activities at the family level are mother and child health, family planning and immunization services. The community health workers can help in imparting nutrition education to the families in their areas.

*At the Community Level*—At the community level, the community health workers will have to obtain information about the nutrition problem in the community and accordingly plan realistic approaches to control the problem. In countries like India, direct intervention measures are implemented like supplementary feeding programs, mid-day school meals, etc. But these will only be temporary solutions. Permanent solutions can only be in the form of some basic measures, which will correct the causes of malnutrition - like increasing the quality and quantity of food and its availability, especially to the people suffering from malnutrition or at the risk of malnutrition. The Applied. Nutrition Program tries to produce different types of protective foods for the community. Also, the Integrated Child Development Services (ICDS) program tries to deliver basic minimum of supplementary nutrition, immunization, health check ups, health education, improvement of water supply, control of infectious diseases, etc., at the community level.

*At the National Level*—At the national level, it is the responsibility of the state to improve the nutritional status of its people. The Report of the joint Food and Agriculture Organization (FAO) /World Health Organization (WHO), Expert Committee on Nutrition suggested various approaches and strategies for action at the national level. It stressed the importance of including food and nutritional planning as a part of the overall socioeconomic development of the country. The FAO was created to look after many areas of world cooperation. The main aim of the FAO is to increase the production of the food in accordance with the growth of the population. Its main concern is to see that food is consumed by the people who need it in sufficient quantities and in right proportions to develop and maintain a better state of nutrition throughout the world. In this context, the government of India has launched several nutritional programs to solve its problem of malnutrition - like the Applied Nutrition Program, Mid-day School Meal Program, National Goiter Control Program, Supplementary Feeding Program, Prophylaxis Against Anemia and Vitamin 'A' Prophylaxis for the Prevention of Blindness, etc.

*At the International Level*—Food and nutrition are International problems. The countries can work in cooperation, especially in times of emergencies like floods, drought, earthquakes, etc., when malnutrition becomes a major problem. There are a number of international agencies like the FAO, United Nations International Children's Emergency Fund (UNICEF), WHO, World Bank, United Nations Development Program (UNDP)/ Cooperative for Resistance and Relief Emergency (CARE) which are working in cooperation and helping the national governments in the world to cope up with the problem of malnutrition.

## PROSTITUTION

Prostitution is one of the oldest forms of business transaction of human beings. It is a very serious social problem effecting individuals, families and the community at large. A prostitute is a person (male or female) who agrees to have sexual intercourse with any person, who offers money for such an act. It is a personal disorganization, which ultimately results in the family and community disorganization also. It is an illegal and promiscuous sexual intercourse, with mercenary basis, in cash or kind with an emotional indifference. All kinds of people may indulge in prostitution like the married and unmarried, men and women, widows and widowers and youngsters. Among all these people, the causes of prostitution may be different. Some of the major causes of prostitution pointed out by sociologist who have studied prostitution are socioeconomic causes, biological causes, psychological causes and religious and cultural causes.

As pointed out earlier, prostitution is not only a personal disorganization but also a family and community disorganization. From the health point of view, prostitution results in serious diseases. Studies of prostitutes show that there is a very high percentage of venereal diseases or Sexually Transmitted Diseases (STD) among them. For example, the spread of syphilis, gonorrhea, HIV/AIDS, through prostitution.

These diseases are life threatening and bad for the life of the society. Therefore, efforts have to be made to control and prevent this problem in the society. Legislative measures can help in the prevention and control of the problem in the society. The government of India passed the Suppression of Immoral Traffic Act (SITA) in Women and Girls in 1956, which was later amended and retitled as Immoral Traffic Prevention Act in 1986. According to this act, prostitution in its commercial form as an organized means of livelihood is banned and punishable. It covers all persons, male or female, who are exploited sexually for commercial purposes.

Besides legislative measures for the control of the prostitution, there can also be other measures like making people aware of the problem and its consequences through sex-education, social aspects of sexually transmitted diseases, publicity and propaganda about the laws, provision of alternate employment opportunities, removal of certain social customs of the society, etc.

## ■ RIGHTS OF WOMEN AND CHILDREN

The Hindu social organization has been dynamic. The status of the women in any society is an indicator of the organization of the society. The status of the Indian women has undergone a number of changes through history. Historically, her position in the Indian society can be studied in the Ancient Times, Medieval Times and the Modern Times.

Generally, the status of the women is studied with reference to the status of the men in the society. Where ancient Indian was concerned, the status of the women was almost equal to that of the men in the society. She enjoyed equal freedom like the man in the society. Women had the freedom to participate in all social, economic, political, religious and educational activities.

But, as changes took place in the society, it is observed that during the Medieval Times her status in the society changed drastically. Gradually, she lost all her freedom to do what she wanted. Her position in the society lowered. Also, with the patriarchal type of families, the domination of the males increased. The equality and freedom, which the woman of the ancient time enjoyed was completely lost. Her position was like that of a slave to the men in the society. It was during this time that a number of evil social customs were also prescribe like child marriage, custom of sati, ban on widow-remarriage, denial of opportunity of education, participation in public life, etc.

The status of the woman in Modern India, during the end of the 19th century started changing gradually. Many of the evil social customs of the earlier period were abolished due to the efforts of social reformers, implementation of social legislation, right to education for all, influence of the West, employment of women. Thus, injustice and discriminatory practices against them reduced. With all these changes, there is a change in the social, economic and political life of the woman. This has brought about a greater awareness of their rights among them.

After Independence, the Constitution proclaimed the fundamental right of women to political and legal equality. The modern Indian women, especially the educated class realized and became more aware of their rights - social, political and economic. Educational and employment opportunities for women also brought about a change in the status of the modern woman. Some of the demands of the modern Indian woman are restriction on child manage, opposition to polygamy, equality of marital rights, right to divorce, abolition of dowry system, rights of inheritance, demands of adoption and maintenance, guardianship and separate residence. The right to better living conditions and the right to health and medical services adopted in the Universal Declaration of Human Rights and the Declaration of the Rights of the Child brought about a change in the position of the child and the women in modern India.

## ■ VULNERABLE GROUPS

### Elderly

The population of the elderly i.e. the 60 plus age is increasing in all societies. This is observed in the population pyramid of the Indian society also. Social changes are taking place in the society as a result of industrialization, urbanization, westernization and modernization. The traditional social values, social structure and economy undergo a change. Thus, the elderly now suffer from a number of familial, social, economic and psychological problems. The result of progress and development of the society is the increasing abuse of the elders of the society.

Abuse of the elderly may be less where the family ties are very strong. The members of the family like the joint family take care of the needs of the elders. The abuse of the elderly may take the form of physical abuse, psychological abuse or economic abuse. The causes for such abuse could be sociocultural factors, psychopathology and dependency, related to social changes.

The problems of the elderly can be solved by proper nursing interventions. The family members must be counseled to take care of the elders at home by giving them the proper love, affection and care and supporting them socially and economically. The family must try to provide a proper environment for them to live a peaceful life up to the end.

The government also should mobilize government and non governmental organizations to provide the care and facilities for the elders, which would give them emotional and social support. A proper provision for economic security through old age allowance, pension, accident benefits, free medical aid, part-time jobs, etc., should be made for the elders. This would ensure that the elders would have sufficient assets and income to manage their life. Counseling and treatment centers should be opened to cope-up with personal and family problems that contribute to abuse. In this way, a better quality of life can be ensured for the elders.

## ■ HANDICAPPED

A handicapped person or a disabled person is one who suffers from a deformity in physical or mental capacity, either by birth or due to an accident. Such a person needs to be given special and attention from the people around him, especially his family members. It is their responsibility to see that he is also provided with the basic necessities for his daily living. Such a person needs more of social, psychological and economic support from people around him.

Today, in countries like India, there is a growing awareness about the problems of the disabled both in the government and the society. They are trying to reach out to the disabled people to enable them to become self-sufficient and independent.

A number of social welfare programs for the benefit of the disabled are being implemented in India at the state and central government levels. Besides these, there are also a number of voluntary agencies running welfare projects for the handicapped. The banks help them with loans at concessional rates. Some public and private enterprises reserve vacancies for the disabled. The government gives them special concessions for travel. Homes for the blind and mentally retarded have been set up to take care of them. There are Braille libraries for the blind run by the government or voluntary organizations. Education of the handicapped is encouraged by giving scholarships to the deserving students.

In India, there are four national institutes for the disabled. They are:
1. National Institute for the Orthopedically Handicapped at Kolkata.
2. National Institute for the Visually Handicapped at Dehradun.
3. National Institute for the Mentally Handicapped at Secunderabad
4. Ali Yavar Jung National Institute for the Hearing Handicapped at Mumbai.

These organizations are centers for the training of professionals, production of educational material and other aids for the handicapped, conducting research in rehabilitation and development of suitable model services for the handicapped.

## ■ MINORITY AND OTHER MARGINALIZED GROUPS

All societies have some kind of stratification based on different factors. This stratification gives rise to minority and majority groups in the society. The minority groups are those which are less in number compared to a majority or a dominate a group in the society. They have an inferior or subordinate position in the society. Thus, they lack the social power as compared to the dominant group. The minority group may be treated with prejudice and discrimination by the dominant group. They may remain excluded from the rest of the society.

A majority or a dominant group is one which is numerically greater in the population of a particular area. They enjoy greater political, economic and social power and a higher status in the society. Therefore, the dominant groups are able to have greater control in the society. They tend to dominate the minority groups. The subordinate position of the minorities in the society denies them equal opportunities to education, occupation and professional advancement.

The concept of minority is usually applied to racial, ethnic, religious, and linguistic groups and sometimes a differentiation is made on physical and cultural factors. The minorities are held in low esteem by the majorities. The majorities dominate the minorities through prejudice and discrimination. Many times, this leads to clashes and conflicts between the two groups in the society.

The constitution of India provides safeguards for the interests of the minorities, weaker sections and the backward classes. National Minority Commission has been set-up by the constitution of India to preserve, protect and promote the religion, culture script and language, rights and interest of the minority groups and to promote the welfare schemes for them. The objective of these provisions is to see that minorities, weaker sections and backward classes are protected socially, economically and politically and help them to acquire their rightful place in the society.

## ■ DELINQUENCY AND CRIME

Crime and delinquency are two major problems especially in the modern societies. The incidence of crime was much less in the primitive societies where the traditions, customs and norms controlled the behaviors of the people. The people followed them strictly. Thus, they acted as strong social controls. But, as the societies started developing, these norms lost their importance for them. This leads to anti-social behaviors in the society. Such anti-social behaviors of people in the society is called as crime. These are generally disapproved by the society. There is a penalty or punishment attached to the crime. Thus, C Darrow defines crime as "an act forbidden by the law of the land and for which penalty is prescribed."

Some of the important causes of crime are the following:
1. Physical and developmental factors like age, sex, physiological defects, race and nativity.
2. Psychological and educational factors like mental deficiency, mental illness, emotional instability and conflicts, educational status.
3. Cultural and environmental factors like family status, marital status, economic status, seasonal aspects, social values, religion, employment, wages, business, customs and traditions, politics and media like TV films, newspapers, etc.

## Juvenile Delinquency

Juvenile delinquency is another major social problem in the modern complex societies. It is an anti-social behavior pattern of children below a specified age according to the law of the state. In short, a juvenile delinquent is a child, generally below the age of 15 or 16, who has committed a crime. Such children cannot be given the same kind of punishment as an adult criminal. There are special juvenile courts and children's homes to take care of such delinquents.

## Causes

Some of the important factors, which are responsible for delinquency are the following:

1. *Social Causes*—Broken homes and families, lack of parental affection and security, quarrels between parents, increase in rates of desertion, separation or divorce, emotional tensions during early age, parental rejection, parental isolation, parental deprivation, illegitimate parenthood and unwanted children, lack of family ties, parental irresponsibility and poverty are some of the social reasons of delinquency.
2. *Physical and Biological Factors*—Physically and mentally handicapped, any sickness and disease, create an inferiority complex leading to anti-social behaviour among children.
3. *Influence of Community*—Institutions, recreation centers, films, commercial amusement, newspapers, magazines, objectionable literature, neighborhood and companionship are also important causes of juvenile delinquency.

Thus, in general it can be said that juvenile delinquency is the result of the social, economic, psychological, biological, environmental and personal factors.

## Prevention and Control

There are two methods for dealing with the problem of juvenile delinquency. They are the preventive method, where the factors leading to delinquency have to be studied and the rehabilitative method, which tries to help those delinquents who have committed a crime to become normal human beings.

Juvenile delinquency may be controlled by taking certain preventive measures like providing the child and the family with proper guidance, providing good recreational facilities, improving the social and economic conditions of living and giving assistance to underprivileged children.

The rehabilitative methods include legislative measures and establishment of institutions to rehabilitate the juvenile delinquents. Some of such institutions established in India are juvenile courts, remand homes, certified schools, auxiliary homes, foster homes, reformatory schools, borstal institutions, fit persons institutions and uncared children institutions.

## ■ CHILD LABOR-CHILD ABUSE

Child is supposed to be the father of man and a citizen of tomorrow. An individual, a boy or a girl, who is below 18 years of age, is legally called a child. Children have become the focus of attention, especially after the year 1979 was proclaimed as the International Year of the Child by the United Nations.

Child labor is any work or employment takenup by a child. It has both social and economic implications. Any child requires physical, intellectual and social inputs to grow and develop properly. This is denied to a child laborer. It affects their health and physical growth. They may be afflicted with diseases resulting from their work and work conditions. Also, the child's behavior patterns would be affected due to work pressure and work conditions. Thus, child labor is directly related to child health and exerts a negative impact on it.

Children are found to be working in different vocations. They are exploited and exposed to hazardous work conditions, with no proper wages for the hours of work. Their conditions of work are very bad. They are made to work in ill-ventilated, ill-lighted, congested and dirty atmosphere resulting in bad health and diseases. It has been found that children suffer from lung diseases, tuberculosis, eye-diseases, asthma, bronchitis and backaches. Some are injured in accidents at the place of work and become unemployable. Many times they are discarded mercilessly by the employers.

## Government Measures and National Policy of Amelioration

The government believes that it cannot wipe out the problem completely. Therefore, it has tried to improve their working conditions like reducing the working hours, ensure minimum wages and provide facilities for health and education. The national policy has three main aims - legal action focusing on general welfare, development programs for child workers and their families and a project based action plan. But, these measures have not been effective in protecting the child laborer. Even today, the child workers do not have a proper shelter, proper food and education. They run the risk of contracting various ailments and skin diseases. They are exploited by parents, employers, police, drug peddlers and are even sexually abused. Therefore, certain principles of policy are to be followed by the state so that children get an opportunity to develop in a healthy manner.

## Causes of Child Labor in India

There are various factors which are responsible for child labor

1. In poor countries like India, low level of earnings of the adult workers, force the children to work.
2. Employers prefer children as they can be controlled easily and they are a cheap source of labor.
3. Family disorganization is a major cause of child labor.
4. *Apathy of the Government*—The government has not taken any concrete steps to eradicate child labor. Though there are laws against the employment of children, they are not enforced strictly.

## ■ CHILD ABUSE

The extent of child abuse is on the increase in the Indian society. In spite of all the planning, welfare programs, legislative measures and administrative actions, it continuous to be a major social problem in the society. The children continue to remain in distress and turmoil. In most families, the parents neglect them, caretakers batter them and in work places employers sexually abuse them. Thus, this problem of emotional, physical and sexual abuse of children in India is on the rise.

According to Burgess, child abuse refers to "any child who receives non-accidental physical and psychological injury as a result of acts and omissions on the part of his parents or guardians or employer." Verbal abuse, threats of physical violence and excessive physical punishment, which do not require medical attention, are also in the definition of child abuse. Child abuse is usually classified into physical, sexual and emotional. Besides these three types, there is also the social abuse.

## Causes of Child Abuse

The major causes of child abuse are adaptational failure or environmental maladjustment (both in the family and work place) mostly on the part of adult perpetrators, like parents and employers, but to some extent on the part of adults responsible for family socialization as well.

## Causes of Physical Abuse

Different scholars have suggested different causes of physical abuse. Some consider psychopathology of the individual perpetrators as the primary cause, while others view psycho-social pathology of families as the main cause. Some others emphasize acute stress.

## Causes of Sexual Abuse

The four causes of sexual abuse are - adjustment problems of the perpetrators, family disorganization, victim's characteristics and psychological disorders of the abusers. The four variables related to sexual abuse are family environment, family structure, individual predispositions and situational factors. The environment in the work place also contributes to sexual molestation.

## Causes of Emotional Abuse

The four important causes of emotional abuse are - poverty, deficient parental control and noncordial relations within the family, maltreatment faced by parents in their own childhood or intergenerational transmission of child maltreatment and alcoholism of parents.

### Effects of Abuse on Children

Bolton and Bolton have identified the possible effects of abuse on children as - physical, sexual, social and emotional. They are self-devaluation, dependency, mistrust, revitalization, withdrawal from people, emotional trauma, deviant behavior and interpersonal problems.

### ALCOHOLISM

Alcoholism is the major social and medical problem. Over the past few years the consumption of alcohol has increased and the age at which people have started drinking has also declined. This is due to the socio-economic and cultural changes. Many times alcohol is viewed as a symbol social status and prestige.

Alcoholism is the excessive consumption of alcohol and getting addicted to it. It starts as an individual problem, which effects the family, the community and the society at large. It effects the individual health and interferes with his social and economic functioning. It may start as an experiment or as a recreation or for relaxation purpose and may end up as compulsive drinking which leads to addiction. The alcoholics may be classified as rare drinkers, infrequent drinkers, light drinkers, moderate drinkers and heavy drinkers.

### Causes of Drinking and Evil Effects of Alcoholism

A number of social, economic, psychological and physical causes may lead to alcoholism. Alcoholism is harmful for the individual as well as the family and the community. It thus becomes a social evil. The continues consumption of alcohol has a number of ill-effects on the individual and destroys his health. It effects the individual physically, mentally and socially. It effects the brain and its efficiency. It may lead to family disorganization, poverty, quarrels, abusive behavior and crime and anti-social activities. The individual may be effected by diseases of the gastrointestinal tract, cardiac problems, blood, muscles, skin, nutrition and reproduction system. Besides these, he may also suffer from psychiatric problems. When an individual tries to decrease his consumption of alcohol, he experiences withdrawal symptoms like tremors, seizures, hallucinations, behavioral problems, occupational problems, etc.

Mass education can play an important role in controlling the problem by bringing about awareness about the problems of alcoholism among the people. De-addiction, detoxification and treatment centres can also help alcoholics.

## ■ SUBSTANCE ABUSE OR DRUG ABUSE

Substance or drug abuse is one of the major problems facing the society. It can be considered as an aberrant behavior, as well as a social problem. As an aberrant behavior, it is regarded as an individual's social maladjustment and as a social problem. Drug abuse is viewed as a widespread condition that has harmful consequences for the society. The concepts of drug, drug abuses, drug dependence, drug addiction and abstinence syndrome are all related. "Drug" is a chemical substance associated with distinct physical and/or psychological effects. Drug abuse alters a person's normal bodily processes or functions. In the medical sense, a drug is a substance prescribed by a physician or manufactured precisely for the purpose of treating and preventing a disease and ailment by its chemical nature and its effects on the structure and functions of a living organism. In the psychological and sociological sense, "drug" is a term used for a habit forming substance, which directly affects the brain or nervous system. According to Jullian Joseph, "a drug is any chemical substance, which directly affects bodily function, mood, perception or consciousness, which has the potential for misuse and which may be harmful to the individual or the society." Some drugs are harmless and are not addictive but some illegal drugs like heroin, cocaine and LSD, or legal drugs like alcohol, tobacco, barbiturates and amphetamines have harmful physical effects on the individual.

"Drug abuse" is the use of illegal drugs or misuse of legal drugs resulting in physical and psychological harm. It includes smoking, ganja or hashish, taking heroin or cocaine and lysergit acid die thylamide (LSD), injecting morphine, drinking alcohol and so on.

"Drug dependence" is the habitual or frequent use of a drug. The "dependence" may be physical or psychological. Physical dependence also known as "addiction" occurs with the repeated use of a drug, when the body has got adjusted to the presence of the drug and will suffer pain, discomfort or illness, if the drug is discontinued.

Body functioning is effected, if the drug is withdrawn and withdrawal symptoms occur.

"Psychological dependence" occurs when an individual comes to rely on drug for the feeling of well-being that it produces.

"Addiction" to a drug means that the body becomes so dependent to the toxic effects of the drug that it cannot do without it. People use drugs to relieve physical and psychological tensions and for mood alteration.

The drugs may be divided into alcohol, sedatives, stimulants, narcotics, hallucinogens and nicotine. Alcohol is used by some people as pleasant and sociable activity, while others take it as a sedative, which calms down the nerves or as a kind of an anesthetic, which reduces the pain of living. The drugs relieve tension and lessen aggressive inhibitions.

Sedatives or depressants relax the central nervous system, induce sleep and provide a calming effect. Tranquilizers and barbiturates fall into this category. As depressants, they depress the actions of nerves and muscles.

Stimulants activate the central nervous system and relieve tensions, treat mild depression, induce insomnia, increase alertness, combat fatigue and excessive drowsiness and lessen excessive inhibitions. The most widely known stimulates are amphetamines, popularly known as "pep-pills", caffeine and cocaine. They are usually taken orally or as injections.

Narcotics, like sedatives, produce a depressant effect on the central nervous system. They produce feelings of pleasure, strength and superiority, reduce hunger, lesson inhibitions and increase suggestibility. Opium, marijuana, heroin, morphine, pathedine, cocaine (all opiates) and cannabis (charas, ganja and bhang) are examples of narcotics.

Hallucinogens produce distortions of perception (seeing or hearing things in a different way than they actually are) and dream image. LSD is a well known hallucinogen, which is a manmade chemical. LSD is usually taken orally but it may also be injected. The effect of an average dose of LSD lasts for eight to ten hours.

Nicotine includes cigarettes, bidi, cigar, snuff and tobacco. It gives relaxation, stimulates the central nervous system, increases wakefulness and removes boredom. Stimulants, depressants, narcotics and hallucinogens are also called as psychoactive drugs.

The causes of drug abuse maybe classified as the following:

1. Psychological causes like relieving tensions, easing depression, reliering inhibitions, satisfying curiosity, relieving boredom, getting kicks, feeling high and confident and intensifying perception.
2. Social causes like facilitating social experiences, being accepted by friends and challenging social values.
3. Physiological causes like staying awake, heightening sexual experiences, relieving pain and getting sleep.
4. Miscellaneous causes like improving study, sharpening religious insight, deepening self-understanding and solving personal problems, etc.

## HIV/AIDS

AIDS (Acquired Immuno-Deficiency Syndrome) is a disease, which is caused by a virus called HIV (Human Immuno-Deficiency Virus). It is a fatal illness, which breaks down the body's immune system, leaving the victim vulnerable to life threatening infections, neurological disorders or unusual malignancies. The infection is such that once infected, it is probable that the person will be infected for life. The term AIDS generally refers to the last stage of HIV infections. The virus can be transmitted to other persons in a number of ways. The basic modes of transmission are sexual transmission, blood transmission and maternal fetal transmission, i.e. mother to child transmission.

The basic approach to control AIDS would be through health education to enable people to make life saving choices. Educational materials and guidelines for prevention should be made widely available. All mass media should be involved in educating the people on AIDS, its nature, transmission and prevention. It touches all aspects of primary health care, including mother and child heath, family planning and education. AIDS control programs should be integrated into the country's primary health care system. The WHO has launched a "Global Programme on AIDS" on February 1, 1987 to provide global leadership and to support the development of National AIDS Programme.

## SOCIAL WELFARE PROGRAMS IN INDIA

Social welfare movement has been gaining ground in India. The Planning Commission set-up by the Government of India in March 1950 formulates the programs of social welfare in the country. The Five Year Plans allocate a huge amount of money for "social welfare". The Department of Social Welfare created in 1964 and elevated to an independent Ministry of Welfare under the central government is responsible for general social welfare. It plans social welfare programs and coordinates welfare services maintained by the government of India, the state governments and the national voluntary agencies.

A Central Social Welfare Board was set up in August 1953 to distribute funds to voluntary social service organizations for "strengthening, improving and extending" the existing activities in the field of social welfare and for developing new programs and carrying out pilot projects. It is an autonomous body. Welfare Boards, consisting of women social workers and representatives of the state governments, have also been constituted and are functioning in all the states.

### Women Welfare

The Department of Women and Child Development, created in 1985, formulates and implements the policies and programs relating to women and child welfare. The various social welfare programs for women and children in India may be broadly categorized as programs for the welfare of women, programs for the welfare of children, composite programs-both for women and children, schemes for the maladjusted groups, schemes for the physically handicapped persons and programs for the welfare of backward classes.

Some of the major programs are social legislation with respect to status of women, marriage and family, divorce, property, dowry system, maternity benefits, insurance schemes, educational programs, employment and income generating programs, hostels for working women, mahila mandals, family life and institutes. Besides these, the government of India has been appointing various communities and commissions from time to time in order to study the problems of women and invite suggestions and recommendations for their solutions. All this shows that today's women in India have better opportunities and avenues in all spheres of life – national, social, economic and political.

## Child Welfare

Children form a major part of the population in India. The major problems of children are illiteracy, exploitation and discrimination. The various schemes of child welfare carried on in India are the constitutional and legislative provisions, which govern the rights of children, Integrated Child Development Services (ICDS) scheme and a number of other important activities and programs for the welfare of children and women.

## Welfare of the Old People or the Aged

The population of the old, i.e. 60 plus age is increasing in India. The aged suffer from a number of familial, social, economic and psychological problems, which make it necessary to have welfare measures for them. The problems have arisen due to the social changes taking place in the society like the disintegration of the joint family, industrialization, urbanization, westernization and the increasing generation gap.

The government tries to help the aged by providing them with certain welfare measures by way of old age pension or provident fund schemes, medical care, housing facilities in the form of old age homes and recreational facilities to relieve them of their loneliness. Besides these, there are also certain voluntary organizations and associations working for the care and welfare of the aged, like Help-Age India and Age-Care India. The central/state governments, municipal bodies, philanthropic societies, voluntary organizations and senior citizens welfare associations have setup homes for the old/elderly citizens.

## Welfare of the Disabled

A disabled person is one who suffers from the loss or impairment of a limb or deformity in physical or mental capability. There is a growing awareness both in the government and in the society to rehabilitate them to make them self-sufficient and independent.

There are four National Institutes in each major area of disability under the Ministry of Welfare. They are the National Institute for the Orthopedically Handicapped at Kolkata, the National Institute for the Visually Handicapped at Dehradun, the National Institute for the Mentally Handicapped at Secunderabad and the Ali Yavar Jung National Institute for the Hearing Handicapped at Mumbai.

There is a rehabilitation council under the Ministry of Welfare, which prescribes the syllabus for the various training programs, recognizes the training institutes and maintains rehabilitation registers. A number of voluntary organizations like the Spastics Society of India, Spastics Society of Northern India, the Spastics Society of Eastern India, the School and Training College for the Deaf at Lucknow, Abhinav Bharti Manovikas Kendra, Kolkata and the Society for the Remedial Education and Counseling for the Handicapped at Kolkata, are all conducting the training of resource persons in their respective fields of disability. They get grants from the Ministry of Welfare. The Ministry of Welfare started the District Rehabilitation Centre Scheme in 1983 for the disabled persons living in rural areas. The Government of India has set up an Artificial Limb Manufacturing Corporation at Kanpur to produce high quality aids and appliances for the handicapped persons. Training facilities for employment are available both in the government and voluntary sectors. About 100 training institutions are providing training in a variety of vocational activities to the handicapped persons. A number of other facilities like bank loans at concessional rates of interest, job reservations in government and public sector undertakings, age relaxation, priority in the allotment of government houses, scholarships for handicapped students, Braille wrist watches and libraries for the blind, organization of sports competitions for the disabled, houses for the mentally retarded and blind children and so on.

The above facilities being provided to the disabled reflect the concern of the central and state governments regarding the problems of the handicapped. But, much more needs to be done to achieve better results and maximum benefits. The Social Welfare Programs in India suffers at the implementation and administrative levels, where the deficiencies need to be rectified to ensure speedy rehabilitation of the disabled.

## Welfare of the Drug Addicts

Drug abuse is another major social problem in India. Along with this problem, is the problem of drug trafficking. The control of drug addiction has to involve identification, referral services, treatment, public awareness, education and rehabilitation, besides controlling the supply of illicit drugs. A number of ministries/departments are concerned with various aspects of the problems of drug abuse like the Ministry of Finance, the Ministry of Health and Family Welfare, the Ministry of Information and Broadcasting and the Ministry of Human Resources Development.

The Ministry of Welfare has taken up a number of welfare programs for the addicts. It has been looking into the educational and social welfare aspects of drug addiction in the society. The Ministry of Welfare has taken up measures towards building awareness and identification, treatment and rehabilitation of drug addicts, through voluntary organizations and the people themselves. A number of de-addiction camps are regularly organized at the community level, with the help of voluntary organizations, providing counseling and treatment facilities to drug addicts.

The government has also passed a number of laws to curb illicit trafficking and smuggling of drugs and preventing drug abuse. All enforcement agencies can take action under the provisions of law. The government has also taken up a number of administrative measures to solve the problem of drug abuse and illicit trafficking. Police measures are taken to check and prevent illicit drug trafficking. For the treatment of drug addiction, facilities have been provided in many hospitals and by voluntary organizations. The Ministry of Welfare provides financial assistance to voluntary organizations for setting up counseling, de-addiction and aftercare centers.

## Welfare of the Underprivileged Sections of Society

The underprivileged sections of the society are the scheduled castes, scheduled tribes and other backward classes. They have been oppressed, suppressed, exploited, humiliated and deprived of equality, liberty and justice in the society. The underprivileged are also known as the downtrodden or deprived classes of the society. The constitution provides protection and safeguards for them, to promote educational, social, economic and political interests and/or removing their social disabilities in the form of representation in legislatures, reservations in services, centrally sponsored schemes of education, aid to voluntary organizations engaged in the welfare of scheduled castes and scheduled tribes.

The tribes were described as aboriginals or backward. But the constitution used the term "scheduled tribes" to describe them. It provides various safeguards for the promotion and protection of the interests of the scheduled tribes. The 20 Point Economic Program of 1986 lays special emphasis on the development of scheduled tribes.

The term backward classes is used to include Scheduled Castes (SC), Scheduled Tribes (ST), Denotified Tribes and Other Backward Classes (OBC). These sections of the community have been facing a number of disadvantages due to the rigid caste system in the Indian society. They have suffered from social, economic and educational disabilities. They have been suppressed and oppressed and denied all opportunities due to the hierarchical caste system present in the Indian society. Therefore, a number of welfare programs schemes and reforms are being implemented by the government to uplift them.

Thus, several plans and schemes are being formulated to solve the social problems existing in the country. Practicable programs of social planning are being formulated and consciously implemented.

### POINTS TO NOTE

1. Social disorganization and social problems—meaning–characteristics
2. Major social problems—causes and remedial measures:
    a. Poverty
    b. Housing
    c. Illiteracy
    d. Food supplies
    e. Prostitution
    f. Rights of women and children
    g. Vulnerable groups—elderly-handicapped-minority and other marginalized groups-child labor and child abuse-delinquency and crime-substance abuse—HIV-AIDS-dowry-unemployment-beggary—alcoholism
3. Social welfare programs in India:
    a. Women and child welfare
    b. Welfare of old/aged
    c. Welfare of disabled
    d. Welfare of drug addicts
    e. Welfare of under privileged section of society

## Social Problems

### NURSING IMPLICATIONS

Understanding the social problems the nurse can act as a help educator, counsellor and alleviate the problems of the people and society. The nurse can also bring about the awareness of the problems and health consequences the various social welfare programs and rehabilitation programs.

### QUESTIONS

1. Define:
    a. Social Disorganization
    b. Social Problem
    c. Illiteracy
    d. Suppression of Immoral Traffic Act (SITA)
    e. Drug abuse and substance abuse
    f. HIV and AIDS
    g. Child labor and child abuse
    h. Poverty
    i. Unemployment
    j. Alcoholism
    k. Beggary
    l. Delinquency and crime
    m. Food supplies
    n. Prostitution
2. Describe the problems of:
    a. Housing in India
    b. Health consequences of poverty
    c. Health effects of alcoholism
    d. Old age
    e. Crime and juvenile delinquency
    f. Health problems of commercial sex
    g. Working women in India
    h. Health problems of untouchables
3. What are the causes of juvenile delinquency?
4. What are the causes of prostitution?
5. Write a note on social welfare programs in India.
6. Bring out the social effects of alcoholism.

# CHAPTER 15

# Social Change

- Meaning Nature and process of social change
- Factors influencing social change
- Cultural change
  - Social change and human adaptation
  - Social change and stress
  - Social change and deviance
  - Social change and health program
- Cultural lag
- Introduction to theories of social change: linear, cyclical, marxian, functional
- Role of nurse as agents of change

Change is the law of nature. The term "change" denotes a difference in anything over a period of time. Social change refers to the changes taking place in the society. Society as already defined earlier is a "web of social relationships". Social relationships are understood in terms of social processes, social interactions and social organization. Thus, the term social change is used to refer to changes in the institutional and normative structure and functions of the society.

## ■ DEFINITIONS

1. *ME Jones*—"Social change is a term used to describe variations in or modifications of any aspect of social processes, social pattern, social interactions or social organization."
2. *S Koenig*—"Social change refers to the modifications, which occur in the life patterns of the people."
3. *Kingsley Davis*—"By social change is meant only such alteration as occur in social organization i.e. structure and functions of society."

4. *HT Majumdar*—"Social change may be defined as a new fashion or mode, either modifying or replacing the old, in the life of a people or in the operation of a society."
5. *MN Jenson*—"Social change may be defined as a modification in ways of doing and thinking of people."

From the above definitions, it can be said that social change is a modification in any aspect of social process.

## ■ NATURE OF SOCIAL CHANGE

The important characteristics of social changes are the following:
1. *Universal Phenomenon*—Social changes occur in all societies at all times. No society remains static. The speed and extent of change may differ from society to society. Some changes may be rapid, some others may be slow.
2. *Community Change*—Social change is a change, which occurs in the whole community and not refers to the change in the life of an individual or a group of individuals, i.e. social change is social and not individual.
3. *Speed of Social Change is not Uniform*—The speed of change is not uniform in all societies. In some societies like the urban communities, the speed of change may be faster than in rural communities.
4. *Nature and Speed of Social Change is Effected by the Time Factor*—The speed of social change is related to the period or time factor and the factors bringing about the change. The social changes that occurred after industrialization were much faster than the changes that occurred before industrialization.
5. *Social Change Occurs as an Essential Law*—Change is the law of nature. Social change may occur naturally due to certain factors or it can be planned by man. The needs and desires of man keep changing. To satisfy his needs and desires, social change becomes a necessity.
6. *Definite Prediction of Social Change is not Possible*—There is no definite law of social change. Therefore, social change cannot be predicted. This is because the exact forms of social relationships, attitudes, ideas, norms and values cannot be predicted.
7. *Social Change Shows a Chain Reaction Sequence*—The social structure of the society consists of a number of interrelated parts.

Thus, a change in one part of the structure of the society results in a chain of changes in the other parts of the society, which in turn beings about a change in the whole way of life of many people. For example, the impact of industrialization on the position of the women in India and other consequent changes in the society.

8. *Social Change is a Result of a Number of Factors*—No single factor can be pointed out as a cause of social change. There are a number of interrelated factors responsible for a social change. This is due to social phenomenon being inter-dependent. Social changes are chiefly those of modification or of replacement i.e. modification of one part influences the other parts and these influence the rest until the whole is involved.

## ■ FACTORS INFLUENCING SOCIAL CHANGE

Social change occurs in all societies at all times. But the rate at which this social change occurs differs from society to society. A number of factors are responsible for this change. The physical, biological, cultural and technological factors are considered as the factors responsible for bringing about social change.

1. *Physical Factors or Geographical or Environmental Factor*—There are a number of geographical or environmental changes taking place on the earth. There are slow geographical changes, as well as occasional changes in nature like a storm or an earthquake or floods. Besides these, there are also the seasonal changes on the earth's surface. These changes in the physical environment bring about social changes. For example, floods may lead to the construction of dams in order to prevent future floods.

2. *Biological Factors*—Biological factors of social change include the plants and animals and the human beings themselves. Man is influenced by the nonhuman biological factors like the plants and animals around him for his survival. The human biological environment includes the factors that determine the numbers, the composition, the selection and the hereditary quality of the successive generations. This human element of the society is constantly changing, which has an effect on the society like the size and composition of the population producing social changes. For example, the phenomenal growth of population may give rise to social problems like unemployment, poverty, low

standard of living, moral degeneration, the level of physical health, malnutrition and creates a demand for more medical and health services.
3. *Cultural Factors*—Culture plays an important role in affecting social changes. As explained earlier, culture is of two types - the material culture and the nonmaterial culture. The material culture is known as civilization. The nonmaterial culture, which is often referred to as just culture consists of our ideas, ideals, beliefs, values, morals, customs, traditions and other institutions. Changes in culture effect social changes. It gives speed and direction to social change. Social changes and cultural changes are closely related.
4. *Technological Factors*—Changes in technology effects social changes. Technology is the application of new discoveries and inventions. It is the systematic knowledge, which facilitates the use of machines or tools. Technology is constantly developing and changing, which effects changes in the structure of the society. It brings about changes in the production technology, changes in the means of communication and transport. These material changes in turn have an effect on the major social institutions like the family, on the economic life, on the state, on religious life, etc. All these changes no doubt, have a major role to play in the development and progress of human civilization. Technology thus, is a means of economic production, which is an end. Ogburn therefore opines that "technology effects the society by changing over environment to which we in turn adapt. The change is usually in the material environment and the adjustments we make with changes often modify customs and social institutions." Based on this principle he put forward his concept of "cultural lag".

## Human Adaptation and Social Change

As observed earlier, change is a law of nature. Social changes keep taking place continuously in all aspects of society. Man, living in this society, gets effected by these changes. He has to therefore adjust himself to these changing conditions around him. He does this by adapting himself to the new conditions. In this way, he will be able to live a happy, better and satisfied life for example. Man has adjusted himself to the changes in the structure of the family from a joint to a nuclear family, changes in the status of women and empowerment of women effecting the family relations. He also adapts himself to the changes in the physical environment around him which lead to social changes.

## Social Change and Stress

Stress is a condition which an individual experiences when there are a number of social changes taking place around him in his life. If he is unable to adjust and adapt himself to the change in society, he will have stress, conflict, problems related to adjustment and psychosomatic diseases. He will be unable to live a stress-free life. This may lead to frustration, depression, conflict, threat and maladjustment, e.g., changes in technology, family structure, unemployment problems, changing status of the women, etc., may lead to stress for an individual.

## Social Change and Deviance

Every society has its own norms to maintain the social order and peace. Social change is the continues process which needs adaptation. Every society has its sets of norms for its people. People do not conform to all the norms all the time. Social deviance is the act of going against the norms of the society. When people do not adapt themselves to social changes, it may lead to social deviance. Social deviance therefore is the act of going against the rules or norms of the society. This disturbs the social order and peace.

## Social Change and Health Programs

Health programs are important for the welfare of the people. They are implemented by the government to protect the society from health problems. Sometimes people unable to adjust themselves to the changing conditions around them. This may lead to a number of health problems in the society, e.g., the Government of India adopted the Family Planning Programme to control the number of birth in order to improve the quality of life of the population, the Pulse Polio Programme, to Eradicate Polio.

## THEORIES OF SOCIAL CHANGE

Sociologists, historians and social anthropologists have proposed a number of theories of social change. These theories explain the direction and cause of social change.

### Evolutionary Theories of Social Change

The evolutionary theories are based on the assumption that societies gradually change from a simple form to a more complex form i.e. society gradually moves to a higher state of civilization in a linear fashion. These theories were influenced by Charles Darwin's Theory of Organic Evolution.

1. Auguste Comte postulated three stages of social change:
    a. Theological stage is the first stage where man believed that supernatural powers controlled and designed the world. He advanced gradually from belief in fetishes and deities to monotheism. This stage gave way to the Metaphysical stage.
    b. Metaphysical stage is the stage during which man tries to explain the phenomenon by resorting to abstractions.
    c. Positive stage is the stage when man considers the search for ultimate causes hopeless and seeks the explanatory facts that can be empirically observed. This implies progress, which according to Comte will be assured if man adopts a positive attitude in the understanding of natural and social phenomenon.
2. Hebert Spencer compared the society to an organism. According to him, society is gradually progressing towards a better state i.e., from a stage of militarism to a stage of industrialism. In its military stage, society was characterized by warring groups, by a merciless struggle for existence while in the stage of industrialism, it is marked by greater differentiation and integration of its parts. This makes it possible for the different groups – social, economic, political and racial to live in peace.
3. *Theory of Deterioration*—According to some social thinkers, man originally lived in a perfect state of happiness in a golden age. Then, gradually deterioration began to take place with the result that man reached an age of comparative degeneration. Thus, according to Indian mythology man has passed through four ages or yugas—*satyuga, tretayuga, dwaparayuga* and *kaliyuga*.

## Cyclical Theories of Social Change

Some social scientists explain social change as a cycle. According to them, human society goes through certain cycles. Society has a predetermined cycle of birth, growth, maturity and decline. History repeats itself. Society after passing through all stages returns to the original stage, when the cycle begins again. In Hindu mythology, satyuga will again start after kaliyuga is over.

Spengler developed the Cyclical Theory of social change. He analyzed the history of various civilizations and concluded that all civilizations, including the Egyptian, Greek and Roman, pass through a similar cycle of birth, maturity and death. According to him, the Western civilization is now on its decline.

Pitrim Sorokin also concluded that civilization fall into three major types namely, the ideational, the idealistic and the sensate. According to him, civilizations alternate or fluctuate between two cultural extremes – the ideational and the sensate. Ideational culture includes those things, which can be perceived only by the mind. It is abstract like religion, faith, truth, etc. The sensate culture stresses those things, which can be perceived directly by the senses. It is practical and materialistic. Too much emphasis on one type of culture leads to a reaction towards the other. Between these two cultures, is the third type i.e. idealistic culture, which is a happy and a desirable blend of the other two, but no society seems to have achieved it as a stable condition.

Arnold Toynbee, a British Historian, maintained that civilizations pass through three stages, corresponding to youth, maturity and decline. The first is marked by a "response to challenge", the second is a "time of troubles" and third is characterized by degeneration or conflict.

## Deterministic Theories of Social Change

According to the Deterministic Theory, there are certain forces, social or natural or both, which being about social change. It is certain forces or circumstances, which determine the course of social change. Karl Marx was of the view that material conditions of life are the determining factors of social change. His theory is known as the Theory of Economic Determination. According to him, human society passes through various stages, each with its own well-defined organizational system. Each successive stage comes into existence as a result of conflict with the one preceding it. This change is due to changes in economic factors like the methods of production and distribution. A change in the material conditions of life brings about changes in the social institutions like the family, religion or state, which in turn effects the socioeconomic relationships. Thus, economic factor is important for all social aspects of life are dependent on it and are almost entirely determined by it.

### Functionalist or Dynamic Theories of Social Change

According to this theory, when change takes place in any one of the elements in the system, it tends to make further changes in other elements, which accommodates the new elements, so that the integration will be possible i.e. the systems exist because of the equilibrium. The social order is balanced. T Parsons and RL Merton explained social change in terms of social equilibrium.

## ■ ROLE OF NURSE AS AGENTS OF SOCIAL CHANGE

Health is an integral part of community development. The standards of health are closely related to the economic and social structure of the community. Health care of the community needs preventive and curative services, which can be provided by the nurse. The health centers deal with health aspects of the individual, family and community for which the services of the nurse are required. The nurse can bring about a change among the people, with her interaction with them at various levels. She can become an effective agent of social change.

> **POINTS TO NOTE**
> 1. Social change–definition–meaning–nature–process.
> 2. Factors influencing social change.
> 3. Theories of social change.
> 4. Cultural change and cultural lag.
> 5. Role of nurses as an agent of social change.

## NURSING IMPLICATIONS

Nurse can be an effective agent of social change in healthcare of the community, since it needs preventive and curative services, which can be provided by the nurse. The nurse can bring about the change in the people by interaction with them at various levels.

## QUESTIONS

1. Define:
    a. Social change
    b. Cultural lag
2. Explain the following:
    a. Technological factor of social change
    b. Consequences of social change
    c. Role of the nurse in bringing about social change
3. Discuss briefly the various factors of social change with suitable examples.
4. Discuss the theories of social change.
5. Write short notes on:
    1. Human adaptation and social change.
    2. Social change and stress.
    3. Social change and deviance.
    4. Social change and health programs.

# CHAPTER 16

# Social Security and Social Work

➤ Social security
➤ Social security legislations in India
➤ Social work

## ■ SOCIAL SECURITY

Social security is the protection given by the society to its members. They are certain public measures against social and economic distresses which man may face during his lifetime, e.g., unemployment, invalidity, disability, injuries and sicknesses, maternity and so on which makes it difficult for him to earn his living. Social security therefore provides for such contingencies and protection of the individuals. Thus, it is provide social protection to the needy people. This is secured through various forms of public assistance, social insurance and preventive health and welfare services. Social security includes economic, social and physical considerations. It includes statutory enactment, social assistance and social insurance. It also includes schemes enforced and regulated by the government or some public authority on its behalf. The benefits generally covered by social security schemes are medical care, sickness benefit, unemployment benefit maternity benefit, invalidity benefit, survivor's benefit and so on.

Social security is given to the needy people in the form of the following:
- *Social insurance*—aims at giving benefit to the insured on compulsory basis in terms of unemployment, sickness and other emergencies.
- *Social or public assistance*—a kind of help which depends upon certain conditions and legalities between workers and the state. It is generally given by the government to the needy irrespective of the causes or circumstances of the need, e.g., the old or blind who

are economically poor it is given in the form of family allowances, unemployment allowances, old age pension, etc.
- *Public service*—those benefit and services which may be provided by the government on a general basis to all members of the group based on age, sex or other consideration, e.g., children allowances and mental health services.

## ■ SOCIAL SECURITY LEGISLATIONS IN INDIA

There are a number of social security legislations covering various aspects of socio-economic life in India. Some of the risks covered under the Social Security Acts in India are:
- *Death:*
  - Workmen's Compensation Act – 1923
  - Employees State Insurance Act – 1948
- *Disablement:*
  - Workmen's Compensation Act – 1923
  - Employees State Insurance Act – 1948
  - Industrial Employment Standing Order Act – 1946 (Medical aid in case of accident).
  - Central Maternity Benefit Act – 1961
  - State Maternity Benefits Act.
  - Employees State Insurance Act – 1948
- *Sickness:*
  - Employees State Insurance Act – 1948
- *Old age:*
  - Payment of Gratuity Act – 1972
  - Coal Mines Provident Fund and Bonus Scheme Act – 1948
  - Employees Provident Fund Act – 1952
  - Assam Tea Plantation Provident and Pension Fund and Deposit Linked Insurance Fund Scheme Act – 1955
  - Seamen's Provident Fund Act – 1966
  - Employees State Insurance Act – 1948

## ■ SOCIAL WORK

Social work is an applied field of sociology. It is an application of sociological knowledge to the problems of society. Social problems are there in every society, social work has now become a profession.

It is a charitable work and service activities taken up either by individuals or groups or voluntary organizations. The three important functions mentioned by the United Nations is that it is the helping and social activity which denotes liaison activity also.

The basic idea of social work is to reduce individual and social problems. It also tries to assists in advancement and welfare of both. The scope of social work therefore is very wide. It includes providing various type of services to the people like children, women, handicapped, destitute, dependents, disabled persons and so on. For this purpose they have a number of programs of social work like public assistance, social insurance, family services, child welfare services, welfare services for handicapped, women welfare services, labor welfare services, community welfare services and international welfare services.

### POINTS TO NOTE
- Social security meaning-types
- Social work-meaning
- Social security legislation in India.

### NURSING IMPLICATIONS
Knowledge of social security gives an idea of economic, social and physical conditions of patients for nurse which will help in their treatment. Knowledge of social work makes the nurse service minded since it helps in social and liaison activities and in reducing individual and social problems. It tries to assist in advancement and welfare of both individual and society. The nurse can be an educator, by making people aware of various social security measures and social work programs.

### QUESTIONS
1. Define:
   a. Social security
   b. Social work
2. Which are different forms of social security legislations in India?
3. What is the purpose of social work?

# Bibliography

1. Park K. Textbook of Preventive and Social Medicine, Banarasidas Bharot Publishers, Jabalpur.
2. Indrani TK. Textbook of Sociology for Nurses, Jaypee Brothers Medical Publishers (Pvt.) Ltd. New Delhi.
3. Shankar Rao CN. Principles of Sociology with an Introduction to Social Thought, S. Chand and Company Ltd. New Delhi.
4. Vidyabhushan and Sachadeva DR. An Introduction to Sociology, Kitab Mahal, New Delhi.
5. Broom L, Selznick P. Sociology Row Peterson and Co. New York.
6. Kingsley Davis. Human Society, the Macmillan Co.
7. Desai AR. Introduction to Rural Sociology in India, Bombay.
8. Ghurye GS. Caste and Class in India. Popular Book Depot, Bombay.
9. Horoton and Hunt. Sociology, McGraw Hill, New York.
10. Johnson HM. Sociology. Allied publishers, Bombay.
11. Kapadia KM. Marriage and Family in India.
12. MacIver and Page CH. Society—an introductory analysis.
13. Kappiswamy B. Social Change in India.
14. Madan GR. Indian Social Problems.
15. Mamoria CB. Social problems and social disorganisation in India.
16. Peter Worsley. Introducing Sociology.
17. Pascual Gisbert. Fundamentals of sociology.
18. Ramanath Sharma. Principles of sociology: Media promoters and publishers, Bombay.
19. Shankar Rao CN. Sociology, vol I and II.
20. Ram Ahuja. Social Problems in India.
21. Srinivas MN. Case in Modern India and Other Essays.

# Index

## A

Accommodation 52, 60
  forms of 54
  methods of 54
  role of 57
Achieved status 160-162
Acquired immunodeficiency syndrome 203, 216
Age distribution 170
Age-pyramid 170
Agricultural occupation 123
Alcoholism 213
  evil effects of 213
Amalgamation 59
Anonymity 87
Anthropology 9
Anticipatory socialization 36
Antyodaya Program 196
Anuloma 116
Applied nutrition program 203
Arbitration 55
Ascribed status 160-162
Asian mongol 166
Assam Tea Plantation Provident and Pension Fund and Deposit Linked Insurance Fund Scheme Act 233
Assimilation 57, 60
Audience 88
  characteristics of 88
  types of 89
Australoid 166
Authority, exercise of 105

## B

Beggary 197
Beliefs 112
Bigamy 101, 115
Biological factors 209, 225
Biological problems 194

Birth rate 99
Blindness, prevention of 203
Blood relationship 85, 104
Bushman 166

## C

Case-study method 13
Caste 126, 141, 148, 151
  interdependence of 149
  panchayat 144
  system 150
    characteristics of 144
    demerits of 148, 149
    features of 144, 149
    merits of 148
    origin of 147
Casteism 149
Caucasoid race 166
Center of Quarrels 108
Central Maternity Benefit Act 233
CH Cooley's Classification of Social Groups 78
Chain reaction sequence 224
Child abuse 210, 211
  causes of 212
Child labor 210
  causes of 211
Child marriage 116
  Restraint Act 118
Child welfare 218
Church 35
City
  community 135
  growth of 137, 138
Civilization 132
Clan, functions of 84
Class 141, 151
  conflict 67
  extremes 134
Coal Mines Provident Fund and Bonus Scheme Act 233

# Index

Community  27, 30
  change  224
  characteristics of  29
  development
    program  128
    project and planning  128, 131
  elements of  29
  influence of  209
  sentiment  29
  size of  29
Competition  61, 64, 69
  forms of  62
  functions of  63
  nature and characteristics of  62
  role of  63
  types of  62
Compromise  55
Conciliation  55
Conflict  65-67, 69
  forms of  66
  nature and characteristics of  66
  negative effects of  68
  positive effects of  68
  role of  68
  types of  66
Conjugal family  104
Conjunctive social processes  50
Consanguineous family  104
Conservatism  124, 125
Control over members  84
Conventional audience  89
Conversion  56
Cooperation  64, 69
  importance of  52
  role of  52
  types of  51
Corporate and personal conflict  67
Crime  208
  higher incidence of  135
Crowd  86
  characteristics of  86
Cultural competition  63
Cultural factors  45, 127, 192, 226
Cultural problems  194
Cultural similarity  59
Cultural system  156
Cultural transmission, instrument of  97
Culture  39, 40, 41, 43, 49, 137
  characteristics of  40
  development of  41
  diversity of  42
  elements of  43
  evolution of  41
  functions of  44
  types of  42
  uniformity of  42
Customs  124, 182
  and fashion  187
  and law  185
  social role of  183
  traditional controls of  112

## D

Death  233
Deliberative group  88
Delinquency  208
Demographic cycle  169
Denotified tribes  221
Deterioration, theory of  228
Developmental socialization  36
Direct cooperation  51
Disabled, welfare of  218
Disablement  233
Dispersed group  87
Dissociative social processes  61
Distinctiveness  180
Divorce  100
Dominance  60
Dowry system  117
Drinking, causes of  213
Drug
  abuse  214
  addicts, welfare of  220
Durkheim's classification  157
Dynamic life  135

## E

Eastern pygmy  166
Economic competition  63
Economic factors  127
Economic functions  97
Economic imbalance  100
Economic independence  99, 112
Economic life, changes in  128
Economic problems  194
Economic provision  95
Education  59, 109, 186
Educational facilities  172
Educational functions  97

Educational levels 137
Emotional abuse, causes of 212
Emotional basis 95
Employees Provident Fund Act 233
Employees State Insurance Act 233
Employment Assurance Scheme 196
Encourages litigation 108
Endogamous family 104
Endogamy 115
Environment 136
Ethnocentrism 83
Exogamous family 104
Exogamous group 84
Exogamy 115, 116, 146
Expenditure, economy of 106
Eye infections 138

**F**

Facilities, lack of 138
Family 94, 136
    and marriage 94
    and nutrition 118
    and parents 34
    disorganization 138
    effects of sickness in 119
    forms of 101
    influence of 118
    joint 103
    large 124
    modern 111
    nuclear 103, 111
    planning 172
    system, importance of 125
    types of 101
    welfare services 113
Fashion 186, 187
    characteristics of 187
    social role of 188
Feeding, restrictions on 145
Fever 138
Filocentric family 100, 112
Folkways 179, 181
    characteristics of 180
    sanction of 180
Food
    and Agriculture Organization 202
    problem 172
    supplies 201
Formalistic school 7
Formative influence 96

Fraternal polyandry 101, 115
Frustration 66

**G**

Gastrointestinal tract disorders 138
Gonorrhea 203
Group 74-76
    feeling 125
    marriage 115
    norms 75, 177
    structure 81

**H**

Handicapped 206
Health 98, 149
    problems 138
    programs 227
Hindu Adoption and Maintenance Act 118
Hindu Marriage Act 117
Hindu Married Women's Rights to Separate Residence and Maintenance Act 117
Hindu Minority and Guardianship Act 118
Hindu Succession Act 118
Hindu Widow Remarriage Act 118
Holtentits 166
Homelessness 133
Homogeneity 123
Housing 200
    problem 172
Human adaptation and social change 226
Human immunodeficiency virus 203, 216
Human race 164
Hypergamy 116

**I**

Ill health 172
Illiteracy 125, 199
Indian Administrative Services 16
Indian caste system 142
Indian marriage and family, legislation of 117
Indian rural life, changes in 126
Indian village, characteristics of 124
Individuals

# Index

collection of 74
personality, development of 107
status of 191
Industrial Employment Standing Order
   Act 233
Industrialization 98, 109
Informal social control 176
Information
   education communication 113
   seeking audience 89
Insecurity promote conflicts 66
Instability 100
Institutions, conflict of 191
Integrated Child Development
   Services 202, 218
   Program 196
Intercaste marriages 116
International conflict 67
Interview method 13, 14
Invulnerability 87
Isolation 60, 70
   absolute 70
   linguistic 71
   organic 70
   partial 71
   physical 71
   societal 71
   spatial 70
   types of 70

## J

Jajmani system 149
Jawahar Gram Samridhi Yojna 196
Joint family 103
   characteristics of 105
   system 104
      demerits of 106, 107
      disintegration of 108
      merits of 106
Juvenile delinquency 209, 210

## L

Labor, advantages of division of 106
Latent conflict 67
Laws 184
   characteristics of 185
Legal state 29
Living, low standard of 172
Local self-government 125
Low mobility 124

## M

Major social problems 194
Major urban problems 137
Marital and sexual relationships, laxity
   in 100
Marriage 101, 114, 136
   and family problems 116
   forms of 95, 114
   restrictions on 146
Mates
   choice of 112
   selection of 95
Matriarchal family 102
Matrilineal family 103
Matrilocal family 103
Mediation 55
Medical
   social worker 12
   sociology 10, 11
Melanesian 166
Members, responsibility of 96
Micronesian polynesian 166
Mid-day School Meal Program 203
Minority 207
Modern family 111
   changes in 98
   problem of 100
Mongoloid race 166
Monogamous family 101
Monogamy 114
Mores 179-181
   conflict of 191
Motivation, source of 63
Mutual assistance and protection
   84
Mutual awareness 74
Mutual rights and obligations 105

## N

National catastrophes 192
National Goiter Control Program 203
National Rural Employment Program
   196
Natural environment 123
Negroid race 166
Neighborhood, importance of 125
Non-essential functions 97
   separation of 113
Non-fraternal polyandry 101, 115
Non-sororal polygyny 101, 115

# Index

Norms 66
    internalization of 36
Nuclear family 103, 111
    features of 112
    structure of 111
Nurse, role of 230
Nursing and health care professions 17
Nutrition, expert committee on 202

## O

Occupation 136
    restrictions on choice of 146
Old people, welfare of 218
Opinion poll method 15
Organization, lack of 88
Other backward classes 221
Over-population, consequences of 171
Overt conflict 67

## P

Parent-youth conflict 99
Patriarchal family 101
Patrilineal family 103
Patrilocal family 103
Payment of Gratuity Act 233
Pedocentric family 100, 112
Peer group 34
People, group of 29
Personal conflict 67
Personality, influence on 75
Physical
    abuse, causes of 212
    factors 209, 225
    mobility 136
    proximity 78
Political
    competition 63
    conflict 67
    factors 127
    life, changes in 128
    organization 85
Polyandry 101, 115
Polygamous family 101
Polygamy 115
Polygyny 101, 115
Population 136, 168
    concentration of 137
    control, need for 172
    development 171
    distribution of 169

    explosion 170
    growth 171
    high density of 133
    low density of 123
    Malthusian theory of 170
Poverty 125, 194
    alleviation programs 196
Pradhanmantri Gramoday Yojana 196
Pratiloma 116
Primary functions 96
Primary groups 78, 81
    characteristics of 78
    importance of 79
    relations 124
    role of 91
Primary institution 125
Primary socialization 35
Prime Minister's Rozgar Yojana 196
Privacy 71
    lack of 108
    problem of 138
Prophylaxis against anemia 203
Prostitution 203
Psychological needs, satisfaction of 79
Psychological problems 194
Public 87
    assistance 232
    characteristics of 87
    service 233

## Q

Questionnaire method 13, 14

## R

Race 164, 166
    determinants of 165
Racial conflict 67
Rapid growth of population, causes for 171
Rational group 88
Rationalization 56
Recreational functions 98
Regional community 132, 139
Regions 139
Religion 35, 112, 124, 137, 179
    importance of 85
Religious function 84, 98
Reproductive and Child Health Program 113

Resocialization  36
Respiratory diseases  138
Rights of women and children  204
Role conflict  159
Rural community  122, 136
　problem of  129
Rural health problems  130
Rural marriage and family  128

## S

Sagotra exogamy  147
Sapinda exogamy  146
Sapravara exogamy  147
Scheduled castes  221
Scheduled tribes  221
School and teachers  34
Seamen's Provident Fund Act  233
Secondary controls  134
Secondary functions  97
Secondary groups  78, 80, 81
　characteristics of  80
　importance of  81
　role of  91
Self-sufficient unit  106
Sex relationships, laxity in  112
Sexual abuse, causes of  212
Sexually transmitted diseases  138, 203
Sickness  233
Similar behavior  75
Skin infection  138
Slums, problem of  138
Social act  157
Social adequacy  16
Social assistance  232
Social change  124, 192, 223-225, 227
　agents of  230
　cyclical theories of  229
　deterministic theories of  229
　dynamic theories of  230
　evolutionary theories of  228
　factors influencing  225
　nature of  224
　speed of  224
　theory of  228
Social class  150
Social competition  62
Social contacts  136
Social control  80, 107, 137, 138, 174
　agencies of  178
　formal  176
　types of  175

Social deviance  138
Social differentiation  141
Social disorganization  135, 190
Social distance  136
Social factors  19, 127
Social groups  73
　characteristics of  74
　classification of  76
Social heterogeneity  133
Social insurance  106, 232
Social interaction  49, 155
Social investigations, methods of  12
Social legislation  110
Social life  128
Social medicine  11
Social mobility  64, 126, 134, 136, 152
　kinds of  152
Social norms  177
Social problems  190, 193
Social processes  48
　forms of  50
Social psychology  8
Social regulation  96
Social relations  136
　restrictions on  145
　web of  73
Social role  158, 183, 188
Social sciences  1, 7
Social security  106, 232
　legislations  233
Social status  160
　types of  160
Social stratification  141
Social structure, nuclear position in  96
Social survey method  12
Social system  154-156
　characteristics of  155
　elements of  157
　parts of  156
　principal types of  156
Social telesis  11
Social values  178
　changes in  193
Social virtues  107
Social Welfare Programs  217
Social work  232, 233
Socialization  30, 43
　adverse effect on  108
　agencies of  34
　agent of  97
　concept of  30

process of 30, 31
stages of 32
types of 35
Society 24, 30, 39, 48, 168
characteristics of 26
elements of 25
hierarchical division of 144
history of 2
segmental division of 144
Sociologist 76
Sociology 1-3, 5, 7-10, 24, 73
importance of 15
nature of 4
scope of 6
uses of 17
Sorokin's classification 157
Sororal polygyny 101, 115
Spatial groups 83
Special Marriage Act 118
Specialistic school 7
Spontaneity 87
Spontaneous origin 180
Stability 75, 79
State Maternity Benefits Act 233
Status 137
Stimulus, provision of 79
Stress 227
Sublimation 56
Substance abuse 214
Super ordination and subordination 56
Supplementary feeding program 203
Suppression of Immoral Traffic Act 204
Swarnjayanti Gram Swarozgar Yojana 196
Swarnjayanti Shahari Rojgar Yojana 196
Synthetic school 7
Syphilis 203

**T**

Technological factors 126, 226
Tertiary cooperation 52

Toleration 56, 59
Towns, growth of 137
Toxicity, chronic 138
Traditions 112, 124
Transcultural society 43
Transport and traffic 138
Tribe, characteristics of 85
Trust and unity, lack of 100

**U**

Uncontrolled reproduction 108
Unemployment 196
United Nations Development Program 203
United Nations International Children's Emergency Fund 203
Unity, sense of 74, 85
Universal phenomenon 224
Urban community 132, 136
features of 133
Urbanization 98, 109

**V**

Venereal diseases 203
Vertical mobility 152
Vices, problem of 138
Village
community 122
features of 123
problem of 129
Viral infections 138
Vitamin A prophylaxis 203
Vulnerable groups 205

**W**

War 66, 193
Western influence 110
Women welfare 217
Workmen's Compensation Act 233
World Bank 203
World Health Organization 202

EU GSPR Authorised Reprsentative
Logos Europe, 9 rue Nicolas Poussin
1700, La Rochelle, France
Phone: +33 (0) 6 67 93 73 78
E-mail: contact@logoseurope.eu

www.ingramcontent.com/pod-product-compliance
Ingram Content Group UK Ltd.
Pitfield, Milton Keynes, MK11 3LW, UK
UKHW021051260426

12086UKWH00012B/403